Nutrition for Brain Health: Fighting Dementia

Third Edition

Laura Town and Karen Hoffman

Omega Press
Zionsville, IN 46077
© 2024 Omega Press

ISBN: 978-1-943414-40-6

Production Credits:
Authors: Laura Town and Karen Hoffman
Publisher: Omega Press
Photos: All credited images used under license from Shutterstock.com

Social media connections:
Laura Town
LinkedIn: https://www.linkedin.com/in/lauratown

Omega Press
Facebook:
https://www.facebook.com/omegabookpublishers/

Omega Press Books

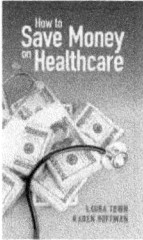

How to Save Money on Healthcare

- People in the United States have over $220 billion in medical debt.
- 20% of Americans have some type of medical debt.
- Over 60% of bankruptcies are related to medical debt.
- 25% of adults have skipped or postponed getting needed health care because of the cost.
- About half of adults would be unable to pay unexpected medical expenses over $500.
- Audiobook, ebook, and paperback available on Amazon.

Long-Term Care Insurance, Power of Attorney, Wealth Management, and Other First Steps

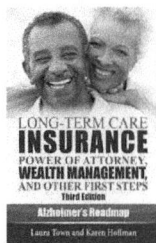

- Getting long-term care insurance earlier is better. Only 20% of people age 50-59 were declined for long-term care insurance, but almost 50% of people age 70-74 were declined.
- Two-thirds of Americans do not have an estate plan, and more than half of people don't know where their parents store their estate planning documents.
- Of those who do have an estate plan, one-third did not include power of attorney documents.
- Audiobook and ebook available on Amazon.

CONTENTS

Introduction

Few things in life are more painful than seeing someone you love slipping away. And few things are scarier than knowing your mind isn't working as it should. My (Laura's) father died of early onset Alzheimer's disease. I suspect that my maternal grandmother also died of early onset Alzheimer's disease. In her case, she was not diagnosed with early onset Alzheimer's, but looking back on it more than 50 years later, it is clear that she, too, had it. When she was diagnosed with "hardening of the arteries" in the 1950s, doctors prescribed electric shock treatments! Fortunately, treatments for dementia patients are more humane now, but we still do not have a cure, and the drugs designed to slow the progression of the disease have produced mixed results.

What we do have, however, is evidence that suggests specific dietary changes and lifestyle changes can help improve memory. Nutritional guidelines based on this evidence can be beneficial to both those wishing to decrease their risk of developing dementia and those hoping to slow progression of the disease. In addition, some dietary changes are specific to preventative means and some are specific to delaying the progression of the disease.

These changes are not easy to make. I am often tempted to drink soda, eat chips, and snack on cupcakes. I have to continuously remind myself that I may pay for these choices in the future and that my children may pay, too, by having to shoulder the incredible burden of caregiving. As you replace the Coke with water, the chips with celery, and the cupcakes with pineapple, remember that you are not only helping yourself; you are also helping your children and the community that must bear the heavy costs of dementia. In 2024, approximately 6.9 million Americans had Alzheimer's disease and health care for these individuals cost an estimated $360 billion dollars. By 2050, it is anticipated that 12.7 million people will have the disease and that care costs will reach almost $1 trillion. And these dollar amounts do not consider the countless hours of unpaid caregiving provided by spouses, families, and friends of individuals with Alzheimer's disease.

A final note about the terms we use in this book. Dementia is a term used to describe a group of symptoms, including memory loss, decline in social abilities, and changes in thinking patterns. The most common form of dementia is Alzheimer's disease, which makes up approximately 60 to 80% of all dementia cases. Vascular dementia and Lewy body dementia are the second and third most common forms of dementia, respectively.

Chapter 1:
Identifying and Addressing Risk Factors

The cause of Alzheimer's disease is not yet understood, but it is believed that a combination of genetic, environmental, and lifestyle factors work together over time to cause the disease to develop. The interaction of these factors varies for every person with the condition, and common risk factors for Alzheimer's disease are described in the following checklist.

Checklist: Risk factors for Alzheimer's disease

☐ **Age.** This is the leading risk factor for Alzheimer's disease. The likelihood of developing the disease increases substantially at age 65. After age 85, the risk of developing the disease is close to one-third.

☐ **Genetics.** Alzheimer's disease tends to run in families, especially in early-onset cases (cases that appear in people younger than age 65). Understanding your family's genetic history of Alzheimer's disease is important.

☐ **Diet and exercise.** Infrequent exercise and an unhealthy diet are both risk factors for developing Alzheimer's disease. This is due to the imbalance or deficiency of nutrients consistent with an unhealthy diet and the extra strain on the body (particularly the heart) associated with the lack of regular exercise. Poor diet can also contribute to the accumulation of "bad" bacteria rather than "good" bacteria in the gut, which further increases the risk for Alzheimer's disease.

☐ **Smoking.** Individuals who smoke are at higher risk for having a stroke, having a heart attack, and developing high cholesterol and blood pressure. All of these factors increase a person's risk of developing Alzheimer's disease later in life.

- ☐ **Alcohol.** Chronic (i.e., long-term) and heavy alcohol use has been shown to increase the risk of developing dementia. The correlation between heavy drinking and Alzheimer's disease is difficult to study because alcoholic dementia and Alzheimer's disease present many of the same symptoms.

- ☐ **Uncontrolled chronic diseases.** Uncontrolled diseases (i.e., diseases that are not adequately controlled through medical treatment) such as diabetes, high cholesterol, high blood pressure, and others can increase the risk of developing Alzheimer's disease.

- ☐ **Lifestyle choices.** Individuals who choose to participate in high-impact sports (e.g., football) or other risky behavior increase their risk of decreased cognitive functioning as time progresses. This results from frequent head injuries, which substantially increase an individual's risk of developing dementia.

- ☐ **Chemical exposure.** A link has been found between an exposure to the pesticide DDT (dichlorodiphenyltrichloroethane) and the development of late-onset Alzheimer's disease. This pesticide has been outlawed in the United States since 1972, but many other countries around the world still use it. Imported fruits, vegetables, and fish could contain high amounts of DDT.

- ☐ **Chronic high stress.** Individuals with frequent high stress are at an increased risk for developing various forms of dementia. Similarly, experiencing stress while a person has Alzheimer's disease has been shown to noticeably accelerate the progression of the disease.

☐ **Depression.** Chronic depression is a risk factor for many diseases, including heart disease and Alzheimer's disease.

Making changes to your eating habits promotes healthy brain activity—even if your risk factors are outside of your control. Many of these changes are easy to incorporate into daily dietary habits, such as increasing daily consumption of coffee to three to five cups, drinking a cup or two of green or black tea, and eating more fruits and vegetables. Other changes are more intensive, depending on your current diet, including ensuring a healthy and balanced diet and participating in a regular exercise routine.

Research has shown that certain additions to a person's diet—like the ones mentioned above—can dramatically decrease the chance of developing dementia, or at the very least slow onset of the disease by years. These changes work to improve both body and brain health. Because being overweight in middle adulthood can increase the risk of developing dementia, some of the same dietary modifications that improve body and brain health can help decrease obesity, which in turn helps prevent the development of dementia.

Nutrition and Obesity

A healthy body mass index may lower the risk of developing dementia, especially Alzheimer's disease. Body mass indexes in the overweight and obese ranges are connected to Alzheimer's disease diagnoses later in life. Therefore, maintaining balanced nutrition and participating in regular exercise throughout life are vitally important. In addition, healthy food choices involving less saturated fats and more foods that help lower cholesterol can be very helpful in preventing or delaying the onset of dementia.

Lowering cholesterol and decreasing saturated fat intake can also help improve your overall health and decrease your risk factors for heart disease and stroke.

BMI	19	20	21	22	23	24	25	26	27	28	29	30	31	32	33	34	35
Height							Weight in Pounds										
4'10"	91	96	100	105	110	115	119	124	129	134	138	143	148	153	158	162	167
4'11"	94	99	104	109	114	119	124	128	133	138	143	148	153	158	163	168	173
5'	97	102	107	112	118	123	128	133	138	143	148	153	158	163	168	174	179
5'1"	100	106	111	116	122	127	132	137	143	148	153	158	164	169	174	180	185
5'2"	104	109	115	120	126	131	136	142	147	153	158	164	169	175	180	186	191
5'3"	107	113	118	124	130	135	141	146	152	158	163	169	175	180	186	191	197
5'4"	110	116	122	128	134	140	145	151	157	163	169	174	180	186	192	197	204
5'5"	114	120	126	132	138	144	150	156	162	168	174	180	186	192	198	204	210
5'6"	118	124	130	136	142	148	155	161	167	173	179	186	192	198	204	210	216
5'7"	121	127	134	140	146	153	159	166	172	178	185	191	198	204	211	217	223
5'8"	125	131	138	144	151	158	164	171	177	184	190	197	203	210	216	223	230
5'9"	128	135	142	149	155	162	169	176	182	189	196	203	209	216	223	230	236
5'10"	132	139	146	153	160	167	174	181	188	195	202	209	216	222	229	236	243
5'11"	136	143	150	157	165	172	179	186	193	200	208	215	222	229	236	243	250
6'	140	147	154	162	169	177	184	191	199	206	213	221	228	235	242	250	258
6'1"	144	151	159	166	174	182	189	197	204	212	219	227	235	242	250	257	265
6'2"	148	155	163	171	179	186	194	202	210	218	225	233	241	249	256	264	272
6'3"	152	160	168	176	184	192	200	208	216	224	232	240	248	256	264	272	279
		Healthy Weight						Overweight						Obese			

Credit: U.S. Department of Health and Human Services

Decreasing Saturated Fats and Cholesterol

Most people have heard of saturated fats and cholesterol, both of which are generally perceived as negative components of a diet. However, both of these are important parts of a person's daily dietary nutrition when consumed in moderation. Saturated fatty acids are the "solid fats" found in many animal-based foods, such as butter, cream, fatty meats, and cheese. Consuming some of these foods is not bad; negative health risks arise when you eat too much food containing saturated fats. Unsaturated fats are considered healthier than saturated fats because they can help improve blood cholesterol levels and are not as likely to lead to weight gain. Unsaturated fatty acids can be found in many plant-based foods and some oils, including olive oil, peanut oil, and corn oil. However, although unsaturated fats are healthier than saturated fats, they should still be eaten in moderation.

A high intake of saturated fatty acids leads to an increase in cholesterol. Two types of cholesterol exist: HDL (high density lipoprotein) cholesterol—or "good" cholesterol—and LDL (low density lipoprotein) cholesterol—or "bad" cholesterol. Bad cholesterol leads to formation of thick, hard plaques that accumulate in a person's arteries, making them inflexible. Inflexible or blocked arteries can inhibit blood flow and increase the risk of developing heart disease. In addition, high levels of bad cholesterol are associated with an increased risk of developing dementia, including Alzheimer's disease. This correlation is hypothesized to be due to several factors, such as decreasing the efficiency of blood flow to the heart, which also decreases blood flow to the brain. If the brain is not receiving enough oxygen-rich blood, then its functionality will decrease and damage can occur. This could speed the development of plaques and tangles in the brain, leading to Alzheimer's disease.

Foods that contain saturated fatty acids include both meat and dairy products. Meat products that are high in saturated fats usually involve fat from the meat itself; for example, fatty beef, pork, and lamb are all high in saturated fat, as is the skin from poultry. Saturated fats are also found in dairy products such as butter, lard, cream, and some types of cheeses. Having some saturated fats in your diet is fine; the problem arises when an excess of them is consumed daily. As long as 5% to 6% or less of your daily caloric intake comes from saturated fats, the amount is not seen as dangerous in most cases. However, if 15% of your daily intake is made up of saturated fats, you are at risk for high cholesterol and thus at an increased risk for Alzheimer's disease and dementia.

Many foods that are high in saturated fats are also high in calories. This essentially means that not only can these foods contribute to high cholesterol, but they can also lead to weight gain. Maintaining a healthy weight is imperative to decreasing your risk for dementia. Individuals with higher body mass indexes have a greater likelihood of developing dementia later in life compared to those with lower body mass indexes. This is likely due to the fact that lower calorie consumption aids in protective brain chemical processes, which help the brain in recovering from injuries or degenerations such as Alzheimer's disease. One way to decrease saturated fat intake and maintain a healthy body weight is to focus on consuming a healthy balanced diet.

Eating a Healthy Balanced Diet

A healthy and balanced diet is an important factor to prevent Alzheimer's disease or dementia. Having a poor diet containing too much of one type of food and not enough of another can damage your brain. This is especially true if you are consuming too much sugar or saturated fat on a daily basis. The best defense, in terms of food and beverage consumption, is to ensure that your diet is both healthy and balanced. This does not mean that you have to give up high-sugar foods all together, but rather that they should be eaten in moderation and in conjunction with other healthy food options.

In order to have a balanced diet, you should have a daily mix of whole grains, refined grains, protein, fruits, vegetables, dairy products, and different types of oils. Each of these food groups should be consumed every day in different amounts, but because they are such broad groups you still have a lot of options. The following checklist discusses some tips for consuming a balanced diet with essential nutrients.

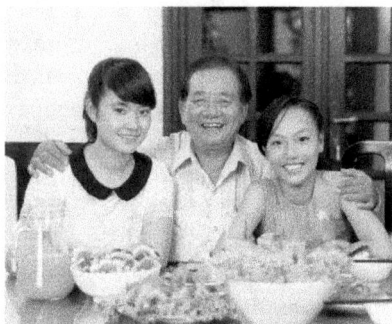

Credit: Dragon Images

Checklist: Tips for a balanced diet

☐ **Grains.** Daily grain consumption should be an even mix between refined grains and whole grains.

8

If your daily recommended grain consumption is 6 ounces, then at least 3 of those ounces should be whole grains, such as whole wheat pasta, brown rice, or buckwheat products.

- **Protein.** Daily protein consumption can be satisfied with several different types of foods, including lean meats, eggs, beans, fish, seafood, soy products, and nuts and seeds.

- **Fruits.** A variety of fruit types should be consumed to get the most nutrients. Raw fruits generally have more nutritional value than store-bought fruit juices.

- **Vegetables.** When choosing vegetables, they should be a mix of red, orange, green, and starchy vegetables.

- **Dairy.** Dairy products can include milk, cheese, yogurt, ice cream, and sour cream. Low-fat or fat-free dairy products are healthier than dairy products containing fat, because much of the fat in dairy products is saturated fat. In addition, the calcium contained in dairy products is more readily absorbed in the presence of vitamin D.

- **Oils.** Oils, while not a food group, are an important part of a healthy diet because they provide essential nutrients. Olive oil is a healthier oil to cook with than vegetable oil or butter. Solid fats, such as lard, butter, and bacon grease, are much less healthy to cook with than the majority of oils.

The nutritional information included on most food products is based on a 2,000 calorie a day diet, but this is not always the healthiest option for all individuals. For example, those who are not very physically active during the day, getting less than 30 minutes of exercise, may only need 1,600 or 1,800 calories a day. Women, in particular, generally

DAILY NUTRITION
BY CALORIES AND FOOD GROUP

1,600 CALORIE DIET
- Grains: 5 oz
- Fruit: 1.5 cups
- Veggies: 2 cups
- Dairy: 2.5 cups
- Protein: 5 oz

1,800 CALORIE DIET
- Grains: 6 oz
- Fruit: 1.5 cups
- Veggies: 2.5 cups
- Dairy: 3 cups
- Protein: 5 oz

2,000 CALORIE DIET
- Grains: 6 oz
- Fruit: 2 cups
- Veggies: 2.5 cups
- Dairy: 3 cups
- Protein: 5.5 oz

2,200 CALORIE DIET
- Grains: 7 oz
- Fruit: 2 cups
- Veggies: 3 cups
- Dairy: 3 cups
- Protein: 6 oz

need fewer calories a day than men. While some people may need less than 2,000 calories a day to maintain a healthy weight or lose excess weight, others may need 2,400 or even 2,600 calories a day to prevent abnormal weight loss. This is generally true of individuals who are active more than 60 minutes a day and currently have a healthy weight range or individuals who have a metabolic disorder that causes unwanted weight loss. One way to determine how many calories you should consume each day is to check an online food plan generator, such as the one at MyPlate, a government resource sponsored by the USDA. Generators such as this one will ask your current weight, height, age, and activity level and then suggest a healthy calorie range based on these factors. Those with health concerns or special dietary needs should consult their doctors about any changes in their regular dietary habits. The graphic on this page gives the suggested daily amounts for each food group based on different calorie requirements.

Portion size is very important when considering a balanced diet. Many people do not realize how small portion sizes should be to adhere to the calorie requirements for a 2,000 calorie or less diet. For example, a hamburger that contains a quarter pound of meat—the typical size of a small hamburger—is 4 ounces of beef (about 28 grams of protein). For a 2,000 calorie a day diet, that one hamburger makes up almost your entire allotment of protein-rich food for the day. The amount of food that is served at restaurants is often much greater than the recommended daily amounts as well. Consider a typical steak dinner at a restaurant. Normally, steaks served at restaurants are between 6 and 12 ounces and come with sides ranging from potatoes and cooked vegetables to a serving of French fries. If you eat the whole steak, you could actually consume up to twice the recommended amount of protein-rich food for the day and a large portion of saturated fat as well. If a baked potato is served with the meal, that is approximately 1 cup or more from your vegetable requirement for the day, and if you add butter and sour cream to your potato, you are again increasing saturated fat consumption. If you also have cooked vegetables on the side, you could get close to 2 cups of vegetables in one meal. All of this is not even including any appetizers, bread, or dessert that was served with the meal. Many restaurants are now required to have calorie counts listed on the menu, so portions are a bit easier to estimate, but it is still good practice to consider how much is being consumed when working to achieve a balanced diet.

Consuming a balanced diet—rather than a diet of all protein and no vegetables or all grains and no protein—allows your body to function at optimal health. Operating at optimal health essentially means that your whole body benefits, including your brain. One common misconception is that the food you eat does not impact your brain health, and thus does not contribute to Alzheimer's disease or dementia. In reality, the food an individual consumes has a direct impact on brain functionality. Foods that are high in sugar or fat slow down brain activity, because they eventually lead to high insulin levels. When the high insulin levels begin to recede, a "sugar crash" occurs, in which you begin to feel sluggish, tired, and unable to process information as quickly as before. If these "crashes" occur frequently, they can cause physical, lasting damage to the memory centers of your brain.

Consuming a balanced diet helps eliminate chances for further damage by supplying the brain with nutrients needed to function at optimal capacity and protect against any harmful chemicals or cell degeneration. A balanced and healthy diet can also help moderate body weight, especially when combined with daily exercise. Engaging in daily physical activities will not only help ensure a healthy body weight, but it can also help prevent early onset of Alzheimer's disease and dementia.

Weight Loss and Dementia

The connection between body mass index (BMI), which is related to body weight, and dementia risk is complex. Most studies indicate that obesity in mid-life is a risk factor for developing dementia later in life. Paradoxically, individuals who see a decrease in BMI later in life are at increased risk for developing dementia; the weight loss is actually a pathological sign that indicates the development of dementia. However, studies have not examined the effect of intentional weight loss (i.e., dieting in overweight or obese individuals) vs. unintentional weight loss (i.e., weight loss associated with pathological conditions) on the risk for dementia. For people who are overweight or obese in mid-life, could intentional weight loss to reach a more healthy BMI be associated with a decrease in dementia risk? This question seems to be unanswered at this point. Weight loss drugs such as Ozempic and Wegovy are currently under clinical trials to determine if they can be used to prevent cognitive decline, but results are not expected until 2025. However, the pathway through which these drugs could prevent cognitive decline is assumed to be through their effects on inflammation, not weight loss.

Exercising

In addition to eating healthy, getting regular exercise helps reduce the risk of dementia. In fact, engaging in regular physical activity can decrease your chances of developing Alzheimer's disease by 45%. Physical activity in

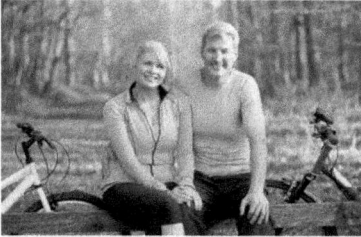
Credit: SpeedKingz

this case does not require running a few miles each day; even mild to moderate activity can help decrease the risk of developing this disease. Exercising 30 minutes a day, 5 days a week can help improve both brain and heart health. Some everyday activities that can contribute to this 30 minutes include swimming, walking, jogging, gardening, cleaning, walking up stairs, doing the laundry, and even grocery shopping. Essentially, any physical activity that works to increase your heart rate will help promote brain health. The reason for this connection between exercise and the decreased risk for Alzheimer's disease is believed to be due to the physical changes caused by exercise.

When an individual increases their heart rate through physical exercise, it causes their blood to pump through the body at a faster rate. This action in turn increases the number of small blood vessels that carry blood to the brain. With an increase in oxygen-rich blood being delivered to the brain, the brain is able to function at an increased capacity. In addition to forming small blood vessels, exercise can increase the number of connections between nerve cells. Nerve cell growth can also be attributed to increased exercise, particularly in the parts of the brain associated with learning and memory. When an individual begins developing Alzheimer's disease or dementia, many of the neural pathways in the brain become damaged or disappear entirely. Studies now show that regular physical exercise can help maintain these neural pathways, thus decreasing the risk for Alzheimer's disease and dementia, or at the very least slowing their progression considerably.

If you have a family history of Alzheimer's disease or dementia or have begun to show early signs of memory loss, exercise could be extremely beneficial. In a study of a group of individuals all genetically predisposed to Alzheimer's disease, those who did not exercise experienced brain shrinkage over the study's time period of a year and a half, whereas those who engaged in physical exercise did not. Scientists studied the area of the brain responsible for short-term and long-term memory, and the individuals who did not exercise experienced a shrinkage of approximately 3% over a year and a half in these areas. Those who participated in mild to moderate exercise showed no change to the memory centers of their brain. Similarly, recent studies indicate that strength or resistance training (e.g., weight lifting) can improve cognitive function in individuals with mild cognitive impairment, potentially even better than aerobic exercises.

Some people hear the word exercise and immediately think of running, jogging, or other activities that are not always enjoyed by most people. However, exercise can be any physical activity that you enjoy doing that increases your heart rate. If you do not like running, or if it is physically painful for you, then consider another activity such as swimming, biking, walking, or skating. You are much more likely to stick with an exercise routine if you enjoy the activity. Similarly, it could be helpful to find a friend to exercise with because this will encourage both of you to continue exercising. You and your friend, or group of friends, could plan to go to the gym a few times a week or plan to take a half hour walk each night. Setting up a regular schedule and including another person in your exercise routine can help make it more enjoyable. Creating goals can also increase your motivation. These goals should be attainable; if you set an unrealistic goal, then you will feel defeated when you do not succeed. Instead, begin with small, attainable goals, and be proud of yourself when you meet them. This success will then help you continue to meet larger exercise goals that you set over time.

Typically, individuals who try to incorporate regular or daily exercise into their routines stop after a week or two, especially if they do not particularly enjoy exercising. If you can stick with an exercise routine for a month, the likelihood of it becoming a habit increases substantially. Creating a habit takes approximately 28 days, at which point the activity becomes routine. If you can commit to 30 minutes of moderate physical activity—such as walking or gardening—for 28 days, the activity will be much easier to continue because it will become part of your daily routine. This exercise will prove beneficial not only to your bodily health but to your brain health as well.

Although exercise in most forms is considered beneficial, high impact sports that have an increased risk of head injury—such as football, hockey, boxing, and rugby—can actually increase a person's risk for Alzheimer's disease and dementia. Repeated head injuries can cause damage to the brain, thus increasing the likelihood of cognitive impairment developing earlier in life. If you or a loved one are at risk for Alzheimer's disease or dementia and choose to begin exercising more regularly, make sure that there is not an increased risk of head injuries associated with that physical activity. Similarly, if you choose to exercise by riding a bike or roller skating, always make sure to wear a safety helmet in case of falls.

Gut and Oral Health

The body has a gut-brain axis and an oral-brain axis that contribute to the overall health of the brain and the body. The gut and the oral cavity both contain a microbiome. These microbiomes are made up of bacteria, and depending on the types of bacteria present, they can either promote inflammation or provide anti-inflammatory properties. The health of these microbiomes and their subsequent inflammatory processes are influenced by what you eat.

Gut Health

New research has found a surprising link between the gut and the development of Alzheimer's disease. The gut, also known as the gastrointestinal system, is home to millions of gut bacteria, called the gut microbiome. "Good" bacteria in the gut promote a healthy gut and anti-inflammatory properties. In contrast, if your gut becomes home for "bad" bacteria, these bacteria can decrease the integrity of the gut barrier, leading to "leaky gut." This leaky gut allows pro-inflammatory molecules to enter the rest of the body and even makes the blood-brain barrier more permeable. When this imbalance of bacteria happens in the gut, it is termed "gut dysbiosis."

Through the gut-brain axis, gut dysbiosis can lead to neurological disorders such as multiple sclerosis, Parkinson's disease, and dementia. In particular, studies have shown that patients with Alzheimer's disease have classical markers for gut dysbiosis. In addition, gut dysbiosis is associated with both beta-amyloid and tau pathologies in Alzheimer's disease. This makes gut dysbiosis a risk factor for developing Alzheimer's disease.

What can cause gut dysbiosis? Many factors can contribute to an imbalance of gut bacteria, including the overuse or misuse of antibiotics, elevated stress levels, lack of sufficient sleep, excessive alcohol consumption, and failure to eat a fresh and balanced diet.

Gut health is highly controlled by what you eat. See the following checklist for foods to eat and foods to limit or avoid to promote gut health.

Checklist: Foods to promote gut health

Foods to eat:

- ☐ Probiotic products (foods or supplements that add good bacteria to the gut)

- ☐ Prebiotic foods (foods that feed good bacteria, such as almonds, bananas, whole grains, flax, cabbage, raw garlic, onion, eggplant, asparagus, honey, raw leafy greens)

- ☐ High fiber foods, such as gluten-free whole grains, fruits, and vegetables

- ☐ Foods high in vitamins A and D [leafy greens (e.g., kale, spinach), yellow and orange fruits and vegetables (e.g., sweet potatoes, carrots, cantaloupe, apricots), red fruits and vegetables (e.g., red peppers, tomatoes), broccoli, summer squash, zucchini, and mushrooms]

- ☐ Fermented foods (e.g., kimchi, sauerkraut, tempeh, miso)

- ☐ Healthy fats (e.g., avocado, extra virgin olive oil)

- ☐ Fish rich in omega-3 fats (e.g., salmon, see *Checklist: Foods that are high in omega 3*)

- ☐ Lean meat, eggs, nuts, and seeds

- ☐ Cultured dairy products (e.g., kefir, yogurt, Greek yogurt)

- ☐ Gut-healthy beverages (e.g., bone broth, coconut milk, water, tea, kombucha)

- ☐ Spices

Foods to limit or avoid:

- ☐ Processed foods, including processed meats, snack foods, and desserts
- ☐ Non-cultured dairy products
- ☐ Foods with emulsifiers (e.g., carrageenans, gums, lecithins)
- ☐ Alcoholic beverages
- ☐ Legumes (e.g., peanuts, beans, peas)
- ☐ Greasy, fatty, spicy, or fried foods
- ☐ Pastries, cakes, cookies, and candy
- ☐ Refined carbs and sugar
- ☐ Soda and energy drinks
- ☐ Artificial sweeteners

Oral Health

Along with gut dysbiosis, poor oral health is linked to Alzheimer's disease. This relationship seems to go both ways. First, poor oral health leads to periodontitis, which is a chronic infectious disease that causes the progressive destruction of supporting tissues of the teeth. Studies indicate that patients with periodontitis have a constant source of bacteria and inflammatory factors that can enter the bloodstream through deep periodontal pockets. These bacteria and inflammatory factors can then cross the blood-brain barrier, causing the activation of microglia and astrocytes in the brain, degeneration of neurons, and deposition of beta-amyloid, a marker for Alzheimer's disease.

Then, once a person starts to show signs of cognitive impairment, including dementia or Alzheimer's disease, the cognitive impairment leads them to forget to complete basic oral hygiene tasks, thus leading to increasingly poor oral health. This cycle leads to increased inflammation, increased cognitive decline, and increased risk of mortality. Along with periodontitis, oral health issues that can lead to cognitive decline include dental caries (cavities), incomplete dentition (having fewer than 28 teeth), and poor chewing ability.

Research on the link between oral health and Alzheimer's disease suggests that good oral health and treatment for periodontitis could help prevent cognitive decline in older adults. Although some studies are conflicting related to the link between oral health and Alzheimer's disease, no studies found that poor oral health is protective against Alzheimer's disease. Instead, poor oral health either had no effect on cognitive decline or increased the risk for Alzheimer's disease. Based on this, maintaining good oral health is a simple way to lower risk for developing Alzheimer's disease.

Checklist: Strategies to improve oral health

- ☐ Brush your teeth twice daily with fluoride toothpaste, brushing all sides of each tooth as well as your tongue. Electric toothbrushes are often more effective than manual toothbrushes for removing plaque.

- ☐ Replace your toothbrush when the bristles become worn.

- ☐ Floss your teeth daily.

- ☐ If you have dentures, clean the dentures every day with mild soap and a soft brush.

- ☐ Watch for signs of gingivitis, or red, swollen, bleeding gums. If you see signs of gingivitis, brush your teeth and floss more frequently and more thoroughly (but not more forcefully).

- ☐ Have your teeth cleaned regularly (every six months) by a dental hygienist to remove calculus, or hardened plaque.

- ☐ Consider asking your dentist or dental hygienist if a fluoride treatment would be right for you.

- ☐ Use a fluoride rinse, such as ACT, and/or an antibacterial mouthwash daily.

- ☐ Drink fluoridated tap water.

- ☐ Don't smoke, vape, or use tobacco products.

- ☐ Don't use cannabis or marijuana. Different forms of cannabis, such as Delta-8, carry many of the same risks as cannabis (Delta-9).

- ☐ Limit sweets and sugary drinks.

- ☐ Consume adequate calcium through foods, drinks, or supplements.

- ☐ If you have periodontitis or other oral infection or disease, seek treatment as soon as possible.

Beverages and Brain Health

When using nutrition to decrease your risk factors for developing dementia, many people overlook the importance of beverages. Coffee, black tea, and green tea all have preventive qualities when it comes to memory loss. Tea and coffee both help memory and brain health due to their natural ingredients. Adding these readily available drinks to your daily routine could prevent you or a loved one from developing Alzheimer's disease or dementia, delay the onset of the disease, or in many cases slow its progression in those who are already experiencing symptoms.

Another beverage that is often discussed when it comes to brain health is red wine. Previous studies have indicated that red wine, consumed in moderation, benefits both heart and brain health. However, these studies are now being called into question. Current evidence suggests that any amount of alcohol consumption, including red wine, is not safe and can lead to adverse effects on health.

Coffee

Many individuals start their morning with a cup of coffee, or they have coffee at some point during the day. Research regarding the negative impacts of coffee has been circulating for years, but a significant amount of research is now being done regarding the connection between coffee consumption, improved memory, and lowered risk factors for Alzheimer's disease, dementia, and general cognitive decline. Drinking between three and five 6-ounce cups of coffee per day can lead to improved memory retention and can significantly reduce your chances of developing Alzheimer's disease. In fact, for some individuals with Alzheimer's disease, coffee consumption can temporarily arrest the progression of the disease for a time, although the disease's progress cannot be halted indefinitely. When drinking caffeinated coffee, it is important to remember that the caffeine content can become detrimental to your health if too much is consumed. Six or more cups of caffeinated coffee per day can cause insomnia, restlessness, and gastrointestinal difficulties.

The reason why coffee can be beneficial is not entirely known, but research suggests that it is not exclusively due to the caffeine content. Caffeine does help people remember facts more effectively, but there are compounds in the coffee itself—both caffeinated and decaffeinated—that are beneficial to memory and brain structure. These compounds appear to be associated with the roasting process and are believed to interact with proteins in the brain.

Tea

Both black and green tea help delay the onset or slow

the progression of Alzheimer's disease and dementia. Black tea is thought to have this effect due to both the caffeine in the drink and the antioxidants in the tea leaves themselves. Similarly, drinking black tea improves memory, information processing, and learning. Generally, drinking one cup of black tea per day can produce these positive changes.

Green tea prevents some processes that could lead to the development of Alzheimer's disease or dementia. In fact, drinking green tea daily results in a 54% reduction in the risk of cognitive decline. The components of green tea reduce plaques that form in the brain; these plaques are thought to contribute to the cognitive decline associated with Alzheimer's disease. The plaques form and stick to the parts of the brain associated with learning and memory. Eventually, they cause damage to those parts of the brain. Researchers have found that green tea actually stops these plaques from forming by preventing them from sticking to healthy neurons in the brain. Additionally, the ingredients of the tea also lead to increased brain cell production and repair of damaged neurons. These new and repaired cells lead to noticeable improvements in memory and learning within a short period of time.

If you or your loved one are at risk of developing Alzheimer's disease or dementia, or already have the disease, drinking one cup of green tea per day could be very beneficial. It is a small change, but it can lead to large improvements. Researchers also found that introducing more green tea did not have negative effects on the brain but rather showed a higher rate of improvement. Therefore, if you or a loved one want to drink two to three cups of green tea per day, it could be even more advantageous to brain health. However, more than five cups per day can cause negative side effects due to the caffeine content.

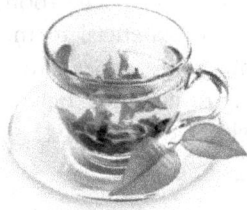

Credit: NataliTerr

In addition to increasing memory, learning, and mental alertness, green tea consumption helps lower cholesterol levels. Drinking one cup of green tea per day for six months results in a decrease in total cholesterol as well as a marked decrease in "bad" cholesterol. As discussed in the section about decreasing saturated fats and cholesterol, high levels of cholesterol increase a person's risk for developing dementia. Therefore, a small change to you or your loved one's daily routine, such as drinking a cup of green tea, could have numerous beneficial effects.

Red Wine

Previous studies indicated that an ingredient in red wine—an antioxidant called resveratrol—can lead to a decrease in plaque formation in the brain. Therefore, drinking one glass of red wine per day was recommended to decrease your risk for Alzheimer's disease or dementia. In contrast, excessive alcohol consumption—four to five glasses of red wine per day or more—can lead to an increased risk of developing Alzheimer's disease or dementia. That leaves the question: At what amount of red wine consumption does it switch from being beneficial to harmful?

Recently, both the World Health Organization and the World Heart Federation published notices that any amount of alcohol consumption, including drinking red wine, carries a risk of harmful effects. In fact, alcohol consumption is linked with 230 ICD-10 diseases, including 40 diseases that would not exist without alcohol. Harmful effects related to alcohol consumption include chronic diseases, liver injury, infectious diseases, digestive diseases, mood and anxiety disorders, and intentional and unintentional injuries.

In particular, alcohol, including beer, wine, and hard liquor, is a known human carcinogen, contributing to the incidence of breast, liver, colon, throat, mouth, and esophagus cancers, among others. This risk for cancer is related to the biological processes the body uses to break down the alcohol, so any amount of alcohol consumption could lead to cancer. Studies have indicated that half of all alcohol-related cancers in Europe are caused by light or moderate drinking. Light drinking is defined as at least 12 drinks in the past year but 3 drinks or fewer per week. Moderate drinking is more than 3 drinks but no more than 7 drinks per week for women and no more than 14 drinks per week for men on average. Note that 5 oz. of red wine is one drink. A standard wine glass holds 12-16 oz. of fluid, so one glass of wine may be equivalent to 2–3 drinks of alcohol.

Red wine is often marketed as being good for your heart. However, studies that support this conclusion were often funded by the alcohol industry, and they did not use large data sets. In addition, they failed to account for other factors that may affect heart health, such as underlying medical conditions and previous alcohol addictions that may cause people to make the decision to abstain from alcohol. Although the data appeared to indicate that red wine was good for heart health, new examination of the evidence does not support this conclusion. In fact, evidence now indicates that alcohol consumption is related to an increased prevalence of cardiovascular disease.

When it comes to brain health, a 2022 study showed that people who drink alcohol have alterations in their brain structure and size, including a reduction in brain volume. These changes are associated with cognitive impairments, and the effects are compounded with each drink. This study found that going from zero to one alcohol unit (half a beer) per day mimicked brain changes associated with half a year of aging. Going from one to two alcohol units (a pint of beer or glass of wine) per day was associated with two years of brain aging. Going from two to three units per day was similar to aging three and a half years. And going from zero to four units per day caused brain changes equivalent to 10 years of aging. This study concluded that although no amount of alcohol is safe, cutting back even one drink per day could have a major effect in terms of brain aging.

Based on this recent evidence, the current recommendation is to abstain from drinking alcohol, including red wine, in order to support your health. Any perceived benefit is vastly outweighed by the numerous potential harmful effects of alcohol. If you find it too difficult to completely abstain from alcohol, limit your alcohol consumption as much as possible. Because the harmful effects of alcohol consumption increase exponentially with each drink, stopping even one drink sooner could decrease your risk of experiencing the harmful effects of alcohol.

Vitamin Deficiencies

Certain vitamins can be extremely important if you are trying to decrease your risk factors for Alzheimer's disease or dementia. The deficiency of some vitamins within the human body can cause adverse symptoms, including memory loss and difficulty connecting ideas. Many lifestyle and health factors can contribute to vitamin deficiencies due to vitamin absorption difficulties, including smoking, certain medications, low stomach acid content, antacids, inflammatory bowel disease (IBD), and Crohn's disease. If vitamins, such as vitamin C and vitamin B_{12}, are deficient for too long, they can cause brain damage and put a person at increased risk for cognitive deficiencies—including Alzheimer's disease and dementia. In addition, vitamin C and vitamin E, when consumed together, help reduce the risk of developing these disorders, or at least slow progression of the disease. In many cases, vitamin deficiencies are best treated by changing your diet to include foods high in those vitamins, but at times doctors will recommend that you begin taking a supplement in addition to dietary modifications.

Vitamin C

Vitamin C is exceptionally important in terms of brain health and cognitive development. Foods that are high in vitamin C not only help keep the immune system strong, they can also help improve memory performance. Many individuals who have Alzheimer's disease and dementia also have a vitamin C deficiency. Although this vitamin deficiency alone will not cause the disease, it could help speed progression and increase cognitive impairment. Increasing your or your loved one's vitamin C intake could help slow the progression of the disease, and it will contribute to your brain and body health in a positive manner. The checklist below highlights some foods that are high in vitamin C.

Checklist: Foods high in vitamin C

- ☐ Acidic fruits (oranges, lemons, limes, grapefruit, pineapple, kiwi, tomatoes)

- ☐ Berries (strawberries, raspberries, blackberries)

- ☐ Dark leafy greens (spinach, kale, salad greens)

- ☐ Green vegetables (broccoli, peas, okra)

- ☐ Cabbage family (cabbage, Brussels sprouts)

- ☐ Melons (cantaloupe, honey dew, papaya, mango, guava)

- ☐ Peppers (red bell, green bell, hot chili peppers)

- ☐ Other (cauliflower, winter squash, sweet potato)

Many supermarkets and health food stores sell vitamin C supplements, but incorporating foods high in vitamin C into your diet is the best approach. These foods are absorbed more efficiently by the body, and they can provide other important vitamins and minerals that have a positive impact on brain health. Some supplements provide doses of vitamin C above the daily recommended amount, and excess vitamin C is typically excreted in the urine. While uncommon, taking too much supplemental vitamin C can lead to digestive issues like diarrhea and nausea in the general population and kidney stones and iron imbalances in people with kidney or liver disease.

Vitamin B$_{12}$

Low levels of vitamin B$_{12}$ can lead to an increased risk for Alzheimer's disease and dementia. This is likely due to the fact that B vitamins are important to neuron health and help maintain stable neuron pathways. When an individual develops Alzheimer's disease or dementia, their neural pathways begin to deteriorate, or shrink, causing less communication between neurons. This eventually results in cognitive decline. Therefore, a vitamin B$_{12}$ deficiency at any point in your or your loved one's life could lead to decreased memory function and should be avoided.

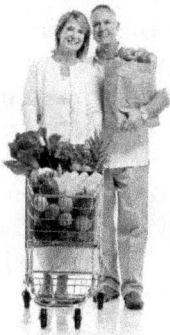

Credit: kurhan

Vitamin B$_{12}$ deficiency is most common in older adults, vegetarians, and vegans. Vitamin B$_{12}$ is found naturally in meat, seafood, and dairy sources, allowing most people to achieve healthy levels of the vitamin within their normal diets. However, if you or your loved one are a vegetarian or vegan—thus not eating meat or dairy products—it can limit the sources of vitamin B$_{12}$ you consume on a daily basis. In these situations, you may need to take vitamin B$_{12}$ supplements or consume sufficient amounts of non-meat or dairy foods that are high in the vitamin. Examples of non-meat foods containing B$_{12}$ include fortified cereals, nutritional yeast, nori, and shitake mushrooms.

Age can also be an important factor in vitamin B_{12} absorption because it becomes more difficult for the body to absorb this vitamin after age 50. Absorption can also be compromised by some medical conditions, such as Crohn's disease, celiac disease, and reduced liver function. If you or a loved one have any medical conditions that reduce absorption of vitamin B_{12}, you should ensure that you are getting enough vitamin B_{12} because this will decrease your risk of developing Alzheimer's disease or dementia. However, taking vitamin B_{12} supplements when you do not have a vitamin B_{12} deficiency does not improve memory or decrease your risk for Alzheimer's disease or dementia. Instead, you should aim to maintain healthy levels of vitamin B_{12} consumption, especially as you progress into your 50s and 60s.

Adults should consume 2.4 micrograms per day of vitamin B_{12}, a level that most people can maintain by eating a regular balanced diet. Women who are pregnant or breastfeeding need to consume more each day to meet their body's needs. If you believe you are suffering from a vitamin B_{12} deficiency, or that you are not consuming enough vitamin B_{12} each day, check with your doctor before taking any supplements or changing your diet. Vitamin B_{12} levels can only be determined through a blood test.

Vitamin D

Optimal vitamin D levels are believed to boost important chemicals that protect brain cells, and vitamin D deficiency can substantially increase the risk of dementia and Alzheimer's disease. Vitamin D is sometimes called the "sunshine vitamin" because the body produces it when it is exposed to the sun's rays. An estimated 61% of seniors are deficient in vitamin D because their sun exposure is limited and vitamin D is only contained in a few foods, including fish, egg yolks, and mushrooms. Some foods that do not naturally contain vitamin D may be fortified with it, including cow and soy milk, orange juice, cereal, and oatmeal.

Vitamin D is actually a hormone that exerts influence on brain function, and research suggests that the risk for Alzheimer's disease and other forms of dementia increases with the severity of vitamin D deficiency. Simple, at-home blood tests can be used to measure vitamin D levels.

There is considerable debate about the ideal vitamin D level and the acceptable daily dose of vitamin D. Recommended doses for adults range from 600 international units per day (iu/day) up to 4,000 iu/day. Because vitamin D is fat soluble, taking too much can cause build up and possible toxicity in the body. Personal vitamin D requirements are based on variables like genetics, sun exposure, and diet. Many vitamin D supplements come in 2,000 iu/day doses of vitamin D_3.

Vitamin D_3 also increases the level of calcium in your blood, but it can raise calcium to unhealthy levels. As a result, it is important to balance vitamin D_3 with complementary supplements that help balance calcium levels. Two common complementary supplements include vitamin K_2 and the mineral magnesium, which we will discuss in the following sections.

Vitamin K_2

For years, vitamin K was associated with blood clotting. However, there are two types of vitamin K, and each type performs a different action in the body. Vitamin K_1 is involved with blood clotting. Vitamin K_2 is associated with calcium distribution in the body.

Vitamin K_2 balances the body's calcium by directing it to areas of the body that need calcium, including the bones and teeth. Without vitamin K_2, calcium can settle in undesirable locations, including the joints, kidneys, blood vessels, and heart. Essentially, vitamin K_2 controls where the calcium you consume winds up.

Vitamin K_2 and vitamin D_3 are often used together. Vitamin D_3 increases the calcium in the blood and vitamin

K_2 tells that calcium where to go, allowing people who take this combination of vitamins to enjoy both a cognitive benefit (from the vitamin D_3) and a bone and tooth strengthening benefit (from the two together).

Experts recommend between 90 and 120 micrograms of vitamin K_2 per day for adults, depending on sex and health condition. The primary natural source of vitamin K_2 is fatty meats; as a result, K_2 supplements may be preferable to natural K_2 consumption. Because vitamin K_1 supports blood clotting, be sure to obtain a doctor's approval before using either a vitamin K_1 or a vitamin K_2 supplement if you or a loved one are taking blood thinners.

Magnesium

Taking magnesium and vitamin D supplements together is more effective at remedying vitamin D deficiency than using vitamin D by itself. Magnesium is involved in the production and use of vitamin D. Magnesium deficiency can cause vitamin D to be stored in an inactive form, resulting in a lack of the expected benefits from vitamin D. In other words, you will not receive the full brain boosting benefits of vitamin D without magnesium. Luckily, magnesium is naturally found in many foods, including those in the following checklist.

Checklist: Foods high in magnesium

- ☐ Avocados
- ☐ Nuts (almonds, cashews, Brazil nuts)
- ☐ Legumes (lentils, beans, chickpeas, peas, soybeans)
- ☐ Tofu
- ☐ Seeds (flax, pumpkin, chia)
- ☐ Whole grains (wheat, oats, barley, buckwheat, quinoa)
- ☐ Fatty fish (salmon, mackerel, halibut)

- [ ] Bananas

- [ ] Leafy greens (kale, spinach, collard greens, turnip greens, mustard greens)

There are also several kinds of magnesium supplements. The most common form found at big box stores is magnesium oxide. This is considered the least effective type of magnesium supplement because it is poorly absorbed by the body.

In addition, some forms of magnesium—such as magnesium citrate—tend to have a laxative effect. As a result, it is recommended to slowly ramp up magnesium supplements to allow the body time to adjust. Magnesium glycinate has less of a laxative effect than other forms and is well absorbed. The recommended daily dose of magnesium for people age 51 and over is 420 milligrams (mg) for men and 320 mg for women.

The graphic on the next page is a quick reference of important vitamins, their daily amounts, and their effects.

Vitamin

BASICS

VITAMIN C

75 to 90 mg of vitamin C each day
aids immunity and memory

VITAMIN B12

2.4 mcg of vitamin B12 each day
keeps neurons healthy

VITAMIN D

600 to 4,000 iu of vitamin D each
day protects brain cells

VITAMIN K2

90 to 120 mcg of vitamin K2 each
day aids calcium distribution

MAGNESIUM

240 to 320 mg of magnesium each
day aids the use of vitamin D

Always talk to your doctor before taking supplements!

Chapter 2:
Eating a Balanced Diet

Eating a balanced diet is important for all individuals, not only those with Alzheimer's disease. However, this may be more important for your loved one with Alzheimer's disease because poor nutrition can result in the worsening of Alzheimer's disease symptoms. A balanced diet contains a variety of foods including fruits, vegetables, grains, protein, and adequate fluids. Fruits and vegetables should make up approximately half of your loved one's daily nutritional intake. This can be in the form of fresh, frozen, or even canned fruits and vegetables. The other half of your loved one's diet should consist of grains and proteins, such as beans, fish, and high fiber fortified grains.

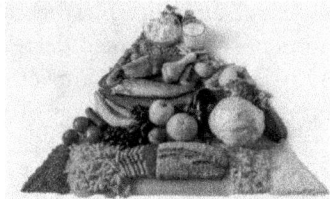

Credit: Mykola Komarovskyy

Brain Healthy Foods

Several foods and food groups can help contribute to increased brain health. Often, this is due to vitamins and antioxidants within the foods that protect brain cells and neural pathways in the brain. Many of these same foods have been proven to produce or stimulate the production of new neurons and pathways. These foods are often referred to as being "brain healthy." Some examples include green leafy vegetables and other dark fruits and vegetables. Foods high in omega 3 fatty acids, such as many types of fish, also promote brain health. These foods help decrease a person's risk factors for Alzheimer's disease and dementia, slow progression of the disease, and in some instances help improve memory function in the mild stage of disease. If you or your loved one are at risk for Alzheimer's disease or dementia, or are in the early stages of the disease, including these brain healthy foods into your diet could be beneficial.

Dark Fruits and Vegetables

Certain foods are more "brain healthy" or "protective" than others, and these can help your or your loved one's memory. These foods reduce damage to brain cells and in some instances increase memory retention and overall brain functioning. Many of these foods are dark-skinned fruits and vegetables, but in particular, spinach, kale, and collard greens are shown to have the most potent and beneficial effects on brain cells. Dark leafy greens, such as spinach, have high amounts of carotenoids and flavonoids, which are nutrients that can help decrease mental decline by almost 40%. For the greatest impact, you or your loved one should eat three or more servings of these foods per day.

The main reason that many of these fruits and vegetables are considered brain healthy is because they contain high amounts of antioxidants. Antioxidants are most commonly found in fruits and vegetables and help prevent or delay cell damage. Some common forms of antioxidants found in brain healthy foods include vitamin C, vitamin E, and beta-carotene. All of these vitamins help delay the onset of Alzheimer's disease and dementia and/or help slow cognitive and physical decline in the earlier stages of the disease. The following checklist highlights fruits and vegetables that are rich in antioxidants and are considered brain healthy.

Checklist: Foods that are high in antioxidants

Vegetables:

☐ Spinach

☐ Kale

☐ Collard greens

- ☐ Brussels sprouts
- ☐ Broccoli
- ☐ Alfalfa sprouts
- ☐ Beets
- ☐ Corn
- ☐ Red peppers
- ☐ Eggplant

Fruits:

- ☐ Blueberries
- ☐ Raspberries
- ☐ Strawberries
- ☐ Blackberries
- ☐ Acai berries
- ☐ Elderberries
- ☐ Cranberries
- ☐ Prunes
- ☐ Raisins
- ☐ Plums
- ☐ Oranges
- ☐ Cherries

Omega 3 Fatty Acids Help Brain Function

Omega 3 fatty acids can help lower your or your loved one's risk factors for Alzheimer's disease and dementia, and they can also help slow the progression of the disease in the early stages. Omega 3s can be found in several different types of foods, but they are mostly found in fish. The reason omega 3s can be so helpful to brain health is because they increase the number of neurons in the brain, produce protective chemicals in the brain, and reduce the formation of plaques and tangles. By consuming foods with this essential fatty acid, you can help improve your overall brain health and decrease cognitive decline.

Checklist: Foods that are high in omega 3

- ☐ Fresh tuna (this should be eaten no more than two times a month because it has a high mercury content)
- ☐ Salmon (wild is best)
- ☐ Mackerel
- ☐ Herring
- ☐ Sardines
- ☐ Trout
- ☐ Anchovy
- ☐ Sea bass
- ☐ Halibut
- ☐ Mussels
- ☐ Shrimp
- ☐ Oysters
- ☐ Grass-fed beef
- ☐ Krill oil and fish oil
- ☐ Flax seeds, or flax seed oil
- ☐ Canola oil
- ☐ Pumpkin seeds
- ☐ Mustard seeds
- ☐ Algae

- ☐ Walnuts
- ☐ Soybeans
- ☐ Tofu
- ☐ Brussels sprouts
- ☐ Cauliflower
- ☐ Green vegetables (both leafy and others)
- ☐ Edamame
- ☐ Fortified products (eggs, milk, cereal, etc.)
- ☐ Oatmeal

You'll notice that seafood, and especially fish, dominates the first half of this list. While eating fish is generally recognized as a healthy choice, mercury poisoning

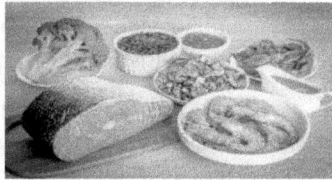

Credit: alexpro9500

is considered a risk with certain varieties of fish. Specifically, king mackerel, marlin, orange roughy, shark, swordfish, tilefish, ahi tuna, and bigeye tuna are all fish that contain high levels of mercury; note that of these fish, only tuna and mackerel are on the checklist above. What does this mean? Potentially, if pregnant women are exposed to high levels of mercury, that could interfere with the brain development of their unborn children. Adults in general, however, have a low risk from mercury exposure. Cooking has no effect on the mercury levels in fish, and mercury isn't something you can taste. Other than mercury levels, PCBs and dioxins present other potential health hazards from eating fish.

The following checklist lays out some food safety facts to consider with regard to fish.

Checklist: Fish and shellfish safety guidelines

☐ Mercury exposure is primarily a risk for pregnant women, women who plan to become pregnant, women who are nursing, and children under the age of six, but most adults have low risk from mercury exposure.

☐ If an adult is concerned about exposure to mercury, limit the consumption of fish high in mercury. From *Checklist: Foods that are high in omega 3*, that means limiting or avoiding the consumption of tuna and mackerel.

☐ Larger fish such as tuna and swordfish are likely to contain higher levels of mercury than smaller fish and shellfish such as squid, scallops, and sardines.

☐ Eat local, and in particular avoid fish imported from countries such as China and Vietnam that have less rigorous management practices for ensuring harvested fish are safe. The US Food and Drug Administration only inspects about 2% of all fish imported to this country.

☐ Buy seafood from trusted sellers with high standards. Fresh fish is safe for purchase only if it is refrigerated or displayed on a bed of ice that is thick and fresh—that is, not melting. All fish should be well-separated in the display.

☐ Use your eyes, ears, and nose to select the best fish. Fish should be springy and resilient to the touch; it should not have an ammonia-like, fishy, or sour smell but should instead smell fresh and mild; and there should be no discoloration or darkening or drying around the edges.

☐ Any fish that will not be used within two days should be stored in a freezer.

- [ ] Thaw fish in the refrigerator overnight or, to thaw quickly, in a plastic bag immersed in cold water or in the microwave on the defrost setting, as long as the defrost cycle does not continue to the point that the fish is no longer icy and pliable.

- [ ] Cook most seafood to an internal temperature of 145°F.

- [ ] Seafood should never be left out of the refrigerator longer than two hours or one hour if the temperature is 90°F or above. For a picnic, pack seafood in ice. For parties, keep hot seafood hot and cold seafood cold.

- [ ] Throw away any shellfish with cracked or broken shells.

- [ ] Remember, higher levels of omega 3s are the potential benefit from eating many types of fish and shellfish. If you are concerned about the health risks of eating fish and shellfish or simply don't like seafood, then try the non-seafood items listed in *Checklist: Foods that are high in omega 3.*

If you or your loved one is in the early stages of Alzheimer's disease or dementia, adding foods rich in omega 3s could help improve memory and slow progression of the disease. These improvements are often seen quickly and can be long-lasting if omega 3 consumption and healthy dietary practices are consistently observed. Eating one to three servings of fish per week has the greatest positive benefit, especially when compared to taking fish oil supplements. Omega 3 supplements can be helpful, but your body will absorb and make use of the omega 3s present in natural sources more efficiently.

Although omega 3 fatty acids help improve memory and boost neuron development, the consumption of a consistently unhealthy and unbalanced diet can negate these positive benefits. For example, if you or your loved one eat three servings of healthy fish or other omega 3-rich foods each week but are otherwise eating foods high in saturated fat, cholesterol, and refined sugars, the omega 3 consumption will not prove beneficial. A healthy, balanced diet is essential to getting the most vitamins and minerals out of foods.

Positive benefits of omega 3 fatty acids have been seen in those with mild Alzheimer's disease and dementia; however, studies have shown that omega 3 consumption has not proved beneficial to those with moderate to severe Alzheimer's disease and dementia. It is best to start these nutritional changes before symptoms arise or at the first signs of cognitive decline. For individuals who carry the E4 allele, a genetic risk factor for Alzheimer's disease, omega 3s have not been shown to help slow progression of the disease or lessen symptoms, even in the earliest stages.

Using Technology to Stay on Track

The food recommendations for a healthy diet are dizzying, and it can be difficult to keep track of what you've eaten and when. Beyond that, it is easy to go into "auto pilot" while eating, especially if you are eating a food you enjoy. When this happens, you may eat far more than a recommended or healthy amount of that food—and fill yourself up too much to eat the right portions of other essential foods.

Tracking what you eat can be a useful way to avoid having these problems. You may choose to keep your tracking simple by jotting down the components of each meal or snack in a small notebook or on a chart taped to the refrigerator. You may also opt to go more technical by using one of the many food tracking apps currently available for smartphones. Examples of these apps include MyFitnessPal, Lose It!, and Cron-o-meter. Although the features of every tracking app differ, they commonly include food diaries that allow you to record what you've consumed, calorie trackers that pair what you ate with its calorie count, and activity logs that allow you to enter in any walking, running, or other exercise you've done. Some include more robust features, too, such as bar code scanners that automatically find a food and its calorie count for you.

If using an app, be sure to look at the fine print and determine whether the app is free or one you must purchase, whether there is a subscription associated with continued use of the app, and whether the company that made the app is trying to sell you a particular product. As with many things related to changing your diet and lifestyle patterns, it is always wise to do your research before making a decision.

Special Nutritional Considerations

If you are caring for a loved one with Alzheimer's disease, it can become more difficult to promote healthy eating habits as the disease progresses. This may be caused by decreased appetite, inability to recognize food, or difficulty swallowing. The following checklist highlights some ways to help your loved one maintain their nutrition, even if eating difficulties are present.

Checklist: Maintaining nutrition with eating and swallowing difficulties

- ☐ Serve bite-sized portions of foods that are easy to pick up and consume, which also makes chewing and swallowing easier.

- ☐ Grind foods, when possible, to make them easier to swallow.

- ☐ Serve soft, nutritious, foods such as applesauce, cottage cheese, canned fruits, and scrambled eggs.

- ☐ Prepare foods that have high nutritional value but can be blended, including fruit or vegetable smoothies, pureed vegetables, and whipped potatoes.

- ☐ Avoid serving foods that could be difficult to chew completely or that pose a choking risk. Some examples of this are raw fruits and vegetables, which could instead be steamed, pureed, or both.

- ☐ Keep meals small and increase their frequency; for example, in place of three large meals a day, try five or six smaller meals throughout the day.

- ☐ Thicken liquids and soups to make them easier to swallow. This can be done by adding unflavored gelatin or food thickeners.

- ☐ If your loved one's sense of taste begins to diminish, try adding natural sweeteners, such as honey, to food to make the food more appealing.

- ☐ Add strong spices to food to enhance its taste, but avoid adding too much salt because it can cause water retention and dehydration.

- ☐ Serve soft fruits and vegetables as snacks, such as bananas, peaches, oranges, and cooked vegetables.

- ☐ Prepare thickened soups and stews that contain large portions of vegetable, dairy, and grain products because this will make it easier to get the most nutrition out of a single, easy-to-eat meal.

- ☐ Serve soups and stews in a mug rather than a bowl so your loved one does not have to struggle with using a spoon.

- ☐ Serve foods that are liquid-based because this can be very helpful in preventing your loved one from becoming dehydrated.

☐ Serve bite-sized pieces of melons, watermelon, and citrus fruits because these fruits contain a lot of water, are nutritious, and are easy to chew.

☐ Prepare meats that are easy to chew, such as pulled pork, chopped meat, or shredded chicken. Steak or thicker cuts of beef or chicken can become tough and difficult to chew and swallow, thus posing a choking risk.

In addition to consuming adequate calories, your loved one needs adequate hydration. Dehydration can lead to confusion, illness, and even pneumonia. Typically, most individuals believe that they need to drink eight 8-ounce glasses of water a day to stay hydrated; while that is not bad advice, staying hydrated is a bit more complex than that. According to the National Academies of Sciences, Engineering, and Medicine, men should drink about 15.5 cups of water a day and women should drink about 11.5 cups of water a day. However, this may be modified by several factors. For example, if you are exercising a lot or it is hot outside, you will need to increase your fluid consumption to replace what is lost through sweating. Water is, of course, the best beverage to consume to stay hydrated, but some individuals have a hard time drinking water. If that is the case for you or your loved one, many foods and beverages contain water and can help keep you hydrated. In addition to water, you can hydrate with coffee, tea, juice, milk, and sports drinks. Some fruits, such as watermelon, are primarily composed of water and can help prevent dehydration. Fruits, such as lemons, limes, oranges, grapes, or grapefruit, can be added to plain water to provide additional flavor. Fruit juices— preferably those made

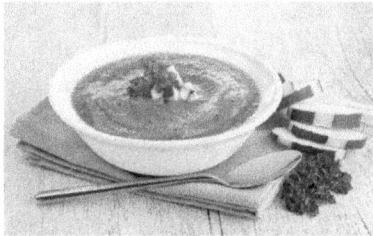

Credit: margouillat photo

from 100% juice with little to no artificial sweeteners—can also be added to water to make it a bit sweeter.

Know What to Expect

Dementia, Alzheimer's Disease Stages, Treatments, and Other Medical Considerations provides answers to the following questions and more:

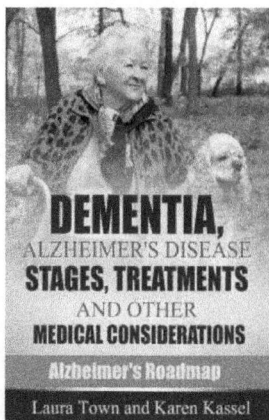

- **What is Alzheimer's disease?** Learn what Alzheimer's disease is, including its characteristics, signs, and risk factors.
- **What can my loved one with Alzheimer's disease expect?** Read detailed descriptions of the stages of Alzheimer's disease, including what patients and caregivers can expect to see at each stage as the disease progresses.
- **What treatments are available?** A survey of prescription medications introduces you to the treatments available to help patients cope with the progression of the disease.
- **What about clinical trials?** Clinical trials are important to finding a cure for Alzheimer's disease, but this book describes the precautions for your loved one to consider before choosing to participate in them.
- **Is there audio for this book?** Yes, you can find the audiobook here: https://adbl.co/2SwzzlA

Chapter 3: Diet Strategies

Numerous diets are popular right now, and it can be difficult to know which might be the best fit for you. It's important to recognize that some diets are just fads and not good long-term choices. It's also important to distinguish between your diet, which is simply what you eat, and a diet, which is a specific approach to eating designed to reach a particular goal. The Department of Health and Human Services (HHS) affirms that maintaining a healthy diet along with exercise can help you maintain a healthy weight, reduce the risk of chronic disease, and improve overall health. But that doesn't mean that any diet will help you achieve these goals. The following checklist describes some current popular diets.

Checklist: Selected popular and healthy diets

☐ The Mediterranean diet focuses on consuming vegetables and fruits (the darker the better), legumes or beans, whole grains, and nuts, with olive oil as the principal source of fat instead of margarine or butter. In this diet, red meat and sweets are consumed rarely; poultry, dairy, and red wine are consumed in moderate portions daily to weekly; and fish and seafood are consumed twice a week.

☐ DASH, or Dietary Approaches to Stop Hypertension, emphasizes foods high in nutrients that lower blood pressure (potassium, calcium, protein, and fiber) such as fruits, vegetables, whole grains, lean protein, and low-fat dairy. It discourages foods high in sodium and saturated fat (fatty meats, full-fat dairy foods, and tropical oils) as well as sugar-sweetened beverages and sweets.

- The MIND diet, which stands for Mediterranean-DASH Intervention for Neurodegenerative Delay, is a combination of the DASH and Mediterranean diets specifically designed to maintain cognitive function.

- The Flexitarian diet is a mostly vegetarian diet that allows the occasional consumption of meat; the vegetarian diet forbids meat but allows dairy products and eggs; and the vegan diet forbids any animal products, including dairy products and eggs. All three of these diets emphasize fruits, vegetables, and grains while making differing allowances regarding meat and dairy.

- The ketogenic diet is characterized by high fat and low carbohydrate intake. By severely limiting carbohydrate intake, this diet promotes ketone production and use for energy rather than simple carbohydrates, which helps burn fat and thus lose weight faster.

- Intermittent fasting, which is not a diet per se but an eating plan or schedule, includes frequent periods with little to no food. Similar to the ketogenic diet, this eating strategy causes the body to switch from using carbohydrates for energy to using stored fat for energy.

- Weight Watchers is focused on losing weight but doesn't put any food off limits. Instead, Weight Watchers assigns a point value to various foods, and people in the program can spend their allotment of points on the foods they want to consume.

- The Mayo Clinic diet uses a Healthy Weight Pyramid that places fruits and vegetables at the bottom of the pyramid, then carbohydrates, protein and dairy, fats, and sweets progressively higher in the pyramid, with a decreased volume of food consumed from each the higher you go.

☐ The Whole 30 diet promotes eating foods with very few ingredients, all pronounceable ingredients, or whole foods with no ingredients listed at all. It encourages moderate portions of meat, seafood, and eggs; a lot of vegetables; some fruit; healthy natural fats; and herbs, spices, and seasonings. The idea behind this diet is to—for 30 days—avoid eating what it deems "problem" foods, including processed snack foods, dairy, legumes, grains, and added sugars, and to avoid consuming alcohol. This is promoted as a detoxification process to heal your gut, restore a healthy gut microbiome, decrease whole-body inflammation, and help you break away from unhealthy patterns of food consumption. After the 30 days, you can slowly reintroduce each food category to identify which foods have a detrimental effect on your body.

These diets are not all the same, but they have similarities. For example, other than the ketogenic diet, they generally favor a low-fat approach focusing on fruits, vegetables, and whole grains and deemphasizing a reliance on meat, poultry, and dairy as dietary mainstays. Many people think of diets as a way to lose weight, but weight loss is only one of the common dietary goals in the following checklist.

Checklist: Common diet goals

☐ Weight loss

☐ Heart health

☐ Diabetes management

☐ Reduction of risk for various other diseases

- ☐ Improved colon health

- ☐ Bone and teeth health

- ☐ Management of food sensitivities, such as sensitivity to gluten

- ☐ Better sleep

- ☐ Improved mood

- ☐ Improved memory

Healthy diets will help you be more mindful of what you eat and have the potential to yield numerous health benefits, though several are more well-suited to promoting brain health than others. It is always best to do your research before embarking on any diet and to discuss the diet and your goals for it with your physician.

Mediterranean Diet

Individuals who live in the Mediterranean region have higher life expectancies than most populations and have a lower rate of individuals with dementia. For this reason, as well as other nutritional factors, the Mediterranean diet is recommended as one way to help lower your risk for dementia. This particular dietary approach can also have a positive effect on those in the early stages of dementia, helping to noticeably slow progression of the symptoms. Additionally, the Mediterranean diet decreases the risk for heart disease and stroke. It also promotes a healthy gut microbiome.

The main component of this dietary approach is eating large portions of fruits, vegetables, whole grains, and legumes. Most, if not all, meals should be made up of these ingredients, with approximately six or more servings of fruits and vegetables per day. In addition, whole grains are very important and should be included in most meals. Fish and seafood are another essential component of this diet, providing protein and omega 3s. Most people who follow the Mediterranean diet consume fish or seafood at least twice a week, if not more frequently. Conversely, red meat should be eaten infrequently, no more than once or twice per month. Poultry, such as chicken and turkey, can be eaten in place of red meat.

In addition to limiting consumption of red meat, the Mediterranean diet also suggests avoiding butter, salt, high fat dairy products, and refined sugars. Butter can be easily replaced in most cases by olive oil, which is a large component of this diet. Extra virgin and virgin olive oil are the healthiest types to use because they contain rich antioxidants. In place of salt, other herbs and spices can be used to add flavor to food as well as to provide additional nutritional benefits. For example, the spice turmeric, often used in curries, helps prevent the formation of plaques in the brain, which could contribute to the development of Alzheimer's disease. High fat dairy products can easily be replaced by skim or fat free options.

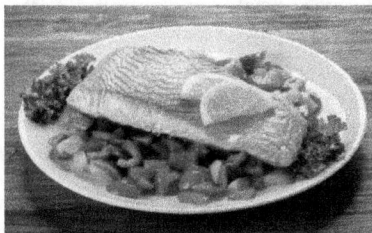
Credit: Jacek Chabraszewski

Nuts, seeds, and red wine are also among the suggested components of the Mediterranean diet. Nuts and seeds are high in both fiber and protein, helping to keep a person full for longer and contributing to a balanced diet. Approximately one handful of nuts per day is recommended, and you should avoid nuts that have been heavily salted or roasted. Some suggestions include walnuts, pistachios, peanuts, almonds, and cashews. Red wine, in moderation, is also recommended a few times a week. However, red wine is no longer recommended for brain health. See the red wine section for more information on this beverage.

DASH Diet

The Dietary Approaches to Stop Hypertension—or DASH—diet focuses on lowering blood pressure by reducing the amount of sodium consumed each day. DASH also promotes eating a variety of foods and nutrients and paying attention to portion sizes. Research has demonstrated a correlation between high blood pressure in mid-life and dementia in later life; as a result, lowering your blood pressure may help reduce your risk of developing dementia.

DASH is a long-term approach to healthier eating rather than a short-term diet plan. It was developed through research sponsored by the National Institutes of Health (NIH) with the goal of lowering blood pressure without medication. It does not involve special foods or complicated recipes; rather, it relies on foods that are easily found in most supermarkets. Beyond decreasing sodium intake and lowering blood pressure, DASH complies with dietary recommendations related to osteoporosis, cancer, heart disease, stroke, and diabetes prevention.

The DASH diet focuses on whole grains, fruits, vegetables, and low-fat dairy products. It also encourages consumption of fish, poultry, beans, and small quantities of nuts a few times each week. Red meat, sweets, and fats are allowed in limited quantities.

The number of calories—and the number of servings of each type of food—allowed each day is based on your age, sex, and level of activity. Calorie ranges fall between 1,600 and 3,000 per day, as described in the following charts. Note that a sedentary activity level involves only light physical activity performed as part of the daily routine, a moderate level involves exercise equivalent to walking up to three miles per day in addition to light physical activity, and an active level involves exercise equivalent to walking more than three miles per day in addition to light physical activity.

Age and Activity Level	Calories Per Day
Sedentary Women	
19 to 30	2,000
31 to 50	1,800
51+	1,600
Moderately Active Women	
19 to 30	2,000 to 2,200
31 to 50	2,000
51+	1,800
Active Women	
19 to 30	2,400
31 to 50	2,200
51+	2,000 to 2,200

Age and Activity Level	Calories Per Day
Sedentary Men	
19 to 30	2,400
31 to 50	2,200
51+	2,000
Moderately Active Men	
19 to 30	2,600 to 2,800
31 to 50	2,400 to 2,600
51+	2,200 to 2,400
Active Men	
19 to 30	3,000
31 to 50	2,800 to 3,000
51+	2,400 to 2,800

The number of servings per day from each food group is based on your calorie needs as determined by the chart. For most people, the servings from the various groups fall into the ranges outlined in the following checklist.

Checklist: Food serving ranges with DASH

Grains

- ☐ 6 to 8 servings per day
- ☐ Whole grain is preferable to refined grain.
- ☐ Avoid using butter, cream, or cheese on grain products.
- ☐ Examples of one serving:
  - ○ 1 slice of bread
  - ○ 1 ounce of dry cereal

o   ½ cup of cooked rice or pasta

Vegetables

- 4 to 5 servings per day
- May be raw or cooked.
- Look for low-sodium options when purchasing frozen or canned.
- Examples of one serving:
  - o   1 cup raw leafy vegetables (salad)
  - o   ½ cup cut up raw vegetables
  - o   ½ cup cooked vegetables

Fruits

- 4 to 5 servings per day
- Leave on edible peels when possible.
- Fresh fruit is preferable and canned fruit or juices should have no added sugar.
- Check with your doctor about citrus fruit and medication reactions.
- Examples of one serving:
  - o   1 medium sized piece of fruit
  - o   ½ cup frozen or canned fruit
  - o   4 ounces of juice

Fat-free or low-fat dairy

- 2 to 3 servings per day
- Regular dairy contains a lot of saturated fat, so stick to low fat options.

- ☐ Cheeses are high in sodium and should be eaten sparingly.

- ☐ If you are lactose intolerant, ask your doctor about over-the-counter treatments.

- ☐ Examples of one serving:

  - o 1 cup of skim or 1% milk

  - o 1 cup of low-fat yogurt

  - o 1 ½ ounces part-skim cheese

Lean meats, poultry, and fish

- ☐ 3 to 6 servings or less per day

- ☐ Choose lean varieties and trim away any skin or fat.

- ☐ Bake, broil, grill, or roast meat rather than frying it in fat.

- ☐ Eat heart-healthy fish like salmon and herring.

- ☐ Avoid deli or luncheon meats, which are high in sodium.

- ☐ Examples of one serving:

  - o 1 egg

  - o 1 ounce cooked meat, poultry, or fish

Nuts, seeds, and legumes

- ☐ 4 to 5 servings per week

- ☐ Phytochemicals in these foods may be protective against cancer and heart disease.

- ☐ Serving sizes are small because calorie content is high.

- ☐ High calorie content also impacts the frequency with which these foods are eaten.

- Examples of one serving:
  - ⅓ cup of nuts
  - 2 tablespoons of seeds or nut butter
  - ½ cup cooked beans or peas

Fats and oils

- 1 to 3 servings per day
- Small amounts of fat are important for nutrient absorption and immune support.
- Too much fat increases the risk of heart disease, diabetes, and obesity.
- Monounsaturated fats are a healthier choice than other fats.
- Examples of one serving:
  - 1 teaspoon vegetable oil
  - 1 tablespoon mayonnaise
  - 2 tablespoons salad dressing

Sweets and added sugars

- 3 to 5 servings or less per week
- When eating sweets, choose those that are fat-free or low-fat.
- Artificial sweeteners should be consumed sensibly.
- Try to reduce added sugar in processed foods.
- Examples of one serving:
  - 1 tablespoon jelly or jam
  - ½ cup sorbet
  - 1 cup lemonade

Sodium

- ☐ 2,300 mg per day maximum

- ☐ When purchasing processed foods, look for options that are sodium free or have no added salt.

- ☐ Use sodium-free spices instead of salt when cooking.

- ☐ Rinse canned foods to remove some of the sodium.

Many of the foods with the highest serving allowances—like grains, fruits, and vegetables—are also high in fiber, potassium, and magnesium. These nutrients are beneficial to lowering blood pressure levels. In addition, many of these foods are also naturally low in sodium, especially in their fresh, unprocessed form.

Although DASH is not a weight-loss focused diet, it can lead to some weight loss by steering you toward healthier food choices. If you are interested in using DASH to lose additional weight, you can select a lower calorie level and follow the portion amounts recommended for that level. Be sure to discuss weight loss goals with your doctor before doing so.

Remember, too, the importance of gradual change when pursuing healthier habits. It is easier to begin something new by adding an extra serving of vegetables here and there and by swapping refined grains for whole grains a little at a time. This will make the change easier on your palate and your digestion, and it can help you avoid feeling deprived of the things you like best. In the long term, your tastes and preferences will change and align with your new, healthier choices.

Additional support and information about DASH—and how to stick to it—are available at nih.gov. There are also several smartphone apps available for the DASH diet. These apps were developed by private companies (not the NIH), and they differ widely in what they offer. Some provide only basic information about DASH, others offer recipes and shopping lists, and still others incorporate food trackers. Some of these apps are free to download and use while others require a monthly subscription. When selecting an app, choose one with the features most important to you and with a fee structure you find acceptable. Keep in mind that the primary focus of DASH is lowering blood pressure, and be wary of any app that claims quick or incredible weight loss as a result of following DASH.

MIND Diet

MIND stands for Mediterranean-DASH Intervention for Neurodegenerative Delay. Martha Clare Morris, a nutritional epidemiologist at Rush University Medical Center, developed the MIND diet specifically to prevent cognitive decline. A study funded by the National Institute on Aging found that the MIND diet lowered Alzheimer's risk. A second paper from Morris's team found that the MIND diet is superior to the DASH and Mediterranean diets for preventing cognitive decline. Since these initial papers, other papers have also been published supporting the usefulness of the MIND diet for supporting brain health and reducing the risk of developing Alzheimer's disease.

The MIND diet is based on two already-established diets, the Mediterranean and DASH diets. The Mediterranean diet was developed from study of the long-term eating habits of Mediterranean people and the observed health benefits of those habits. The DASH diet was developed from clinical trials developed by the National Heart, Lung and Blood Institute (NHLBI). It's also consistent with the recommendations of Dietary Guidelines for Americans developed by HHS. The MIND diet focuses on brain-healthy foods such as berries and green, leafy vegetables; it's consistent with the Mediterranean and DASH approaches, just with a particular focus on specific foods that encourage brain health. The following checklist outlines some MIND diet facts.

Checklist: MIND diet facts

☐ The MIND diet combines the Mediterranean and DASH diets with the specific goal of reducing age-related dementia and a decline in brain health.

☐ The MIND diet emphasizes particular foods:

   ○ Green, leafy vegetables (kale, collards, spinach, lettuce); at least 6 servings a week (such as a salad daily)

   ○ Other vegetables; at least 1 serving a day

   ○ Berries, blueberries in particular; ½ cup serving at least twice a week

   ○ Nuts for snacks; at least 5 times a week

   ○ Whole grains; at least 3 servings a day

   ○ Poultry; at least twice a week

   ○ Fish; at least once a week

   ○ Olive oil for cooking (labeled "extra virgin," not "light;" stored in a dark or opaque bottle because exposure to light is bad for olive oil)

☐ Foods deemphasized in the MIND diet because of their negative effect on cognitive health include:

   ○ Butter or margarine

   ○ Cheese

   ○ Whole dairy products such as whole milk

   ○ Red meat

   ○ Fried foods

   ○ Sweets

☐ This diet may be costlier than some others because items like berries tend to be more expensive.

☐ This diet does not focus specifically on losing weight, but just because that isn't the goal, that doesn't mean you will not lose weight. The foods the MIND diet promotes are not fattening.

☐ You don't need to watch your calories with this diet. Eat until you are full, and then stop.

Plant-Based Diets

Although diets such as the Mediterranean, DASH, and MIND diets are considered plant-based diets because they recommend reduced consumption of animal products, they are not strictly vegetarian or vegan. A vegetarian diet restricts animal products, focusing on the consumption of vegetables, fruits, whole grains, legumes, nuts, and seeds. Vegetarians may also consume limited animal products, such as dairy products and eggs, but they do not consume meats from animals. In contrast, vegan diets avoid all forms of animal products, including dairy products and eggs.

Studies with a vegetarian diet indicate that a vegetarian diet may slow the progression of cognitive decline for patients with Alzheimer's disease. However, a vegan diet has not yet been tested for its effects on cognitive function. One complication with vegetarian and vegan diets is that people who follow these diets can still consume foods that do not support brain health, such as sugar-sweetened beverages, desserts, deep-fried vegetables, and chips. The more you eat of these foods, the less you are supporting your own brain health. In fact, individuals who followed a plant-based diet but consumed higher amounts of unhealthy plant-based foods had faster cognitive decline than those who consumed healthy plant-based foods. The success of plant-based diets for reducing the risk of dementia depends on constant adherence to these diets over decades as well as the types of plant-based foods consumed, genetic variability, and differences in lifestyle factors.

Older adults, including those with cognitive

impairment or Alzheimer's disease, must be careful about switching to a vegetarian or vegan diet. Older adults may require a certain intake of animal-derived products, especially meats, in order to meet their protein needs. In addition, long-term vegan diets may lead to deficiencies in vitamin B_{12} and vitamin D, which may lead to the development and progression of Alzheimer's disease. If you want to follow either of these diets, you will need to make sure you consume adequate nutrients that are normally fulfilled by animal-based products, including protein and certain vitamins.

Ketogenic Diet

A ketogenic diet is characterized by high fat and low carbohydrate intake. The body typically uses carbohydrates, or simple sugars, as its primary source of energy. However, when the body runs out of carbohydrates to convert into energy, it breaks down stored fat, which produces ketone bodies. These ketone bodies are then used by the body for energy.

Studies indicate that a ketogenic diet increased cognitive assessment scores in ApoE4-positive patients with mild Alzheimer's disease, and it also improved cognitive function in patients with mild cognitive impairment or mild to moderate Alzheimer's disease. A ketogenic diet may decrease neuroinflammation, reduce free radicals, and reduce amyloid plaque formation, all of which contribute to a reduced risk of developing neurodegenerative diseases such as Alzheimer's disease. However, more studies are needed to understand the link between the ketogenic diet and Alzheimer's disease.

One drawback of a ketogenic diet is that individuals often do not regulate the type of fat they consume, often choosing to take in fatty meats, bacon, cheeses, butter, and other foods high in saturated fat. This can lead to detrimental effects on the cardiovascular system. Instead, experts recommend focusing on healthier fats to maintain brain and cardiovascular health, such as extra virgin olive oil, salmon, avocado, and nuts and seeds.

One option for following a ketogenic diet is the Modified Mediterranean-ketogenic diet (MMKD), which aims for 5–10% carbohydrates, 60–65% fat, and 30% protein. As is emphasized in the Mediterranean diet, protein sources should be low in saturated fats, such as fish and lean meats. In addition, fat consumption should focus on healthy fats, such as extra virgin olive oil. This diet also promotes the intake of fruits, vegetables, and whole grains as sources of carbohydrates rather than processed grains and sweets. Studies indicate that the MMKD can modulate the gut microbiome and metabolites that are associated with improved biomarkers of Alzheimer's disease. It can also improve cognitive function and everyday functioning.

Intermittent Fasting

Individuals who want the beneficial effects of using ketones for energy without cutting out carbohydrate consumption may choose to implement intermittent fasting. Intermittent fasting requires the individual to go long periods without food, such as alternate day fasting (water-only intake every other day), time-restricted fasting (food intake restricted to 6-12 hours each day), or a 5:2 diet (eating only 500–700 calories for 2 days each week). The periods of fasting should be long enough to switch to a metabolic state in which ketones and free fatty acids are used as the primary source of energy.

Studies indicate that intermittent fasting has positive effects on dementia, including reduced inflammation, better neuron signaling and growth, and reduced insulin resistance in the brain. In particular, alternate day fasting may delay the onset and progression of Alzheimer's disease and Parkinson's disease. Intermittent fasting has been linked to improvement in many diseases, including obesity, diabetes, cardiovascular disease, cancer, immune diseases, and neurodegenerative disorders. However, many individuals also experience harmful side effects with extended or too frequent fasting periods, such as gallstones and increased risk of mortality from cardiovascular disease. More studies are needed to fully understand the link between intermittent fasting, cardiovascular health, brain health, and cognitive function.

Barriers to Diet Success and Fad Diets

In spite of the proven benefits of a nutritious diet—including the Mediterranean diet and DASH—many people struggle with various barriers to successfully follow the diet they choose. Some diets are easier to follow than others, and a lot of that has to do with individual factors. Assess the barriers in the following checklist carefully to find a diet that presents you with the fewest barriers to success.

Checklist: Potential barriers to starting a successful diet

- ☐ Too expensive
- ☐ Not easy to follow
  - ○ Complicated rules
  - ○ Too much calorie counting
  - ○ Too much serving size counting
  - ○ Not enough recipes/too few menu plans
  - ○ Uses uncommon ingredients that are hard to find
  - ○ Restrictions too narrow or too vague
  - ○ Lack of eating out choices
- ☐ Effort of compliance with the diet

o Lack of time

o Poor cooking skills

o Low motivation

o Allergies/aversions to recommended foods

o Needing to cook for others

o Frequent travel

□ Low diversity of foods and flavors in the diet

□ Past failure with sticking to a specific diet

□ Past failure to lose weight when dieting

A diet might also lack basic nutritional soundness, but in this case, that's not a barrier, that's an indication that the diet itself is not good. Carefully considering which diet is right for you is complicated because you should never consider many fad diets in the first place. A fad diet may seem good at first, but if it doesn't include a sound nutritional plan, it could make you feel worse over time. It could even be really dangerous. At the very least, a fad diet won't likely produce any long-term positive effects even if it doesn't actually harm you. You can spot a fad diet by looking for the signs in the following checklist.

FAD DIETS

VERSUS

SAFE DIETS

DETERMIINING IF A DIET IS SOUND

Fad diets rely on a single study or testimonials.	Safe diets are well researched and peer reviewed.
They eliminate food groups they deem "bad."	They limit some foods but do not eliminate them.
They require you to purchase a special product or vitamin.	They require you to purchase food from the grocery store.
They claim that exercise is unnecessary.	They recognize the need for both diet and exercise.

Checklist: Signs of fad diets

- ☐ The diet promises a quick fix with unbelievable-sounding claims that seem too good to be true. If something seems too good to be true, then it probably is too good to be true.

- ☐ The diet relies on a single study or on testimonials (personal stories from people who claim to have used the diet). Safe diets tend to be supported by a lot of research that has been "peer reviewed," meaning the research has been checked out and approved by other experts.

- ☐ The diet relies on research that is in the very early stages or that has produced mixed results. No fad diet based on this type of research will admit that the research is sketchy. Read all you can about any research cited to determine whether you can trust it.

- ☐ The diet calls specific foods or entire food groups "good" and "bad." Typically, safe diets recommend more of something or less of something, but they don't eliminate anything altogether. Vegan and vegetarian diets do eliminate meat and/or dairy, but they recommend substitutes for these foods that provide the nutrients that people normally get from meat and dairy.

- ☐ Following the diet requires buying a special product, such as an herb, vitamin, or supplement. A good diet should only require a trip to the grocery store to buy food. You don't need miracle products.

- ☐ The diet dismisses the need for exercise or claims to provide all the benefits of exercise. A healthy, nutritional diet is only part of maintaining overall health.

If you're unsure about the soundness of a diet you are considering, think about it in light of the information in the quick reference graphic on the previous page and discuss it with your doctor.

Chapter 4:
Pillars of Brain Health

Although there is no cure for dementia, research on other cultures and healthy individuals has revealed new insights into protecting our brains and promoting their health. Brain health is a fairly new concept, but it is consistently being studied and analyzed for clues to help end the scourge of dementia. The Cleveland Clinic has identified six pillars of brain health based on brain health research, as outlined in the following checklist. In architecture, a pillar is a support for a structure. Typically, several pillars are needed to provide proper support; removing any of the pillars weakens the structure as a whole. The same concept applies here. Each of the Cleveland Clinic pillars supports brain health. Removing even one—for example, medical health or sleep and relaxation—weakens your overall brain health. The other pillars still contribute something to your brain health on their own, but they are much stronger together than they are if you focus on only one or two while ignoring the others. What is even more important about these pillars is that they don't just help your brain—they help your whole body. If you concentrate on all of these pillars, you will feel better, think better, be less tired, spend less time being sick, and do more.

Checklist: Cleveland Clinic pillars of brain health

- ☐ Physical exercise

    - ○ Aerobic exercise, such as running, swimming, or biking, builds endurance while also fostering new brain cell growth and preserving existing brain cells.

    - ○ Strength training strengthens both muscle and bone and also boosts brain power, concentration, and decision-making skills.

- Flexibility training improves energy and posture and reduces risk of injury.

- Balance training helps prevent falls and improves overall mobility.

□ Food and nutrition

- Limit red meat.

- Eat fish or walnuts, flaxseeds, and soybeans.

- Eat plenty of fruits and vegetables.

- Eat dark chocolate and use spices like turmeric, cinnamon, and ginger.

- Drink coffee or tea.

- Drink red wine in moderation, or swap out red wine for red grape juice to get the beneficial effects of resveratrol without the harmful effects of alcohol.

- Eat whole grains rather than processed grains.

- Eat eggs in moderation.

- Cut down on sugar and salt.

□ Medical health

- Control risk factors for brain disease such as diabetes, obesity, and hypertension.

- Keep blood pressure and weight in a healthy range.

- Take medication as prescribed.

□ Sleep and relaxation

- Prevent depression.

- Improve mood and overall outlook.

- Manage stress.

☐ Mental fitness

    ○ Build your "brain reserve" to improve adaptability and resist damage to the brain.

    ○ Learn new things to improve cognition.

    ○ Appreciate fine art.

    ○ Play brain-stimulating games such as crossword puzzles or chess.

☐ Social interaction

    ○ Stay connected with other people to reduce stress, combat depression, and enhance intellectual stimulation.

    ○ Enjoy spending time with loved ones.

    ○ Share hobbies and interests through volunteering or joining clubs.

    ○ Get and love a pet.

Nearly all of these pillars involve a lifestyle approach to health. One advantage of lifestyle approaches to preserving or extending cognitive function is that, as in the case of physical and mental exercise, they can have other benefits beyond simply aiding in the prevention of Alzheimer's disease and other forms of dementia. Another advantage is that lifestyle changes are up to you; in other words, they are primarily under your control.

This does not mean lifestyle changes are easy to implement in your own life. Many people struggle with exercise, eating healthy, and sleeping well for a variety of reasons. So, what can you do about it? In general, working on these health domains is like setting and meeting any other goal. The following checklist gives you some general pointers for setting health goals related to the six pillars.

Checklist: Setting health goals

- [ ] A classic approach to setting goals is using the SMART system. SMART is an acronym for the following elements of goal setting:

  - o Specific: The goal should be specific, meaning that it should be something like "I want to do strength training three times a week" and not just "I want to exercise."

  - o Measurable: A goal that is measurable has a concrete means of measuring when it has been attained. "I want to do strength training three times a week, 20 minutes at a time, for three months" is measurable. You know for sure whether you've done it. Did you only do strength training once or twice a week and usually only for five or ten minutes? If so, you didn't meet the goal.

  - o Attainable: An attainable goal is realistic. "I will exercise for two hours every day" is probably not realistic or attainable if you are busy and you don't currently exercise. You have to build up to a goal like that, and spending that much time exercising every day is something you probably won't realistically ever do. But maybe you can identify three times each week when you can exercise for 20 minutes at a time. That's a more realistic start, and then you can build from there.

  - o Relevant: If the goal doesn't help you in some way—if it lacks relevance to your needs or desires—then it doesn't really make sense. For example, doing strength training for your brain health doesn't mean you have to become someone with huge, rippling muscles who can juggle barbells. It just means you work on improving your body's strength. It doesn't have to be for show; it only has to be for you.

o Time bound: Putting your goal on a schedule makes it easier to achieve. If you are prone to procrastination and are always putting things off, having a schedule to meet can help keep you honest and on track. Remember, though, your schedule has to be realistic.

☐ Get started creating a SMART goal by making sure that what you want to do meets all of the SMART criteria. For example: "I want to eat a meatless dinner three times a week for the next two months."

o This is specific: "Eat a meatless dinner."

o It's measurable: "Three times a week."

o It's attainable: You absolutely should be able to plan three meatless dinners a week.

o It's relevant: Brain-healthy diets emphasize eating a lot of fruits and vegetables and reducing intake of red meat.

o It's time bound: "For the next two months."

☐ Write the goal down. This makes it real. Tell someone about it: a spouse or other partner, another family member, or a friend. This will help motivate you.

☐ Break it down. What do you need to do to achieve this goal? Look up recipes? Decide where to buy produce? If meatless dinners are new to you, you might browse the Web looking for good recipes as a starting point. To keep this attainable and relevant, look for recipes for meals you'll actually eat, that don't involve hard-to-find ingredients, that won't cost too much money, and that will be enough food for you and anyone who will eat with you. Also, don't feel like you need to go full vegan right from the start; choose vegetarian recipes with dairy products you like (butter, milk, or cheese). When you've found three recipes for things you think you'll like, decide which store near you has the best produce section for your needs.

- ☐ Plan things out. You've identified recipes to try and the store where you will shop for produce. Now, what's your first step? Go to the store on a particular day at a particular time. What's your next step? Cook the meals on particular days at particular times. If you need to, put all of this in a calendar. For example, you may choose to shop on Sunday afternoons and cook meatless evening meals on Monday, Wednesday, and Friday.

- ☐ Be prepared for mistakes. Maybe you mess up, and you don't get to the store on Sunday. You skip the Friday meal and go out to eat with friends. That's okay; just try to get back on track. Remember, however, that if you continually struggle to meet a goal, you may need to rethink it. It may be better to start with just one meatless meal, not three.

- ☐ Celebrate when you meet a goal. Maybe when you meet your goal each week, you go out with your partner to a movie or go bowling or dancing. Have fun with your goals. They don't need to be a chore.

Chapter 5: Dos and Don'ts of Brain Health

To make the pillars of brain health work to your advantage and help them be easier to follow, it might be useful to think of them in terms of dos and don'ts, as outlined in the following checklist.

Checklist: Brain health dos and don'ts

Do:

☐ **Eat healthy.** Try following a routine like the MIND diet (which combines two popular and healthy diets, DASH and the Mediterranean diet), focusing on fruits and vegetables (the more varied and colorful the better), and taking in enough of the proper nutrients (especially omega 3 fatty acids, vitamin E, vitamin D, B-complex vitamins, and folic acid).

☐ **Exercise.** This definitely means aerobic exercise, but not just that. Strength, flexibility, and balance training are all necessary forms of exercise, too. Building your body builds better brain health.

☐ **Manage stress.** You can't eliminate stress from your life, and some stressors can be positive motivators. But you can and should eliminate unnecessary stressors from your life that cause aggravation, and developing useful ways for dealing with stress can affect your mood and your brain health. Some of the best ways to manage stress include doing other things on this list, like exercising, eating a healthy diet, and connecting with others. But you can also take charge of your stress by following the four A's of stress management while always—first and foremost—staying positive:

o   Avoid stress when you can.

o   Alter the stressful situation if you can.

o   Accept situations you can't change.

o   Adapt to stressors when you can.

☐   **Sleep.** This can be difficult for many people, but seven to eight hours of sleep is essential to long-term brain health. People struggle with sleep for many reasons. Here are some things you can do if you have trouble sleeping:

o   Develop a set routine, going to bed at the same time each night and going into relaxation mode around the same time every night to get in the right frame of mind and body.

o   Reading a book, listening to quiet music, turning the lights down low, and soaking in a warm bath are good types of relaxation. Looking at electronic screens—TVs, computers, smartphones, or tablets—can make it more difficult to get to sleep and aren't the best when bedtime is approaching.

o   Prepare your bedroom by ensuring it's at a comfortable temperature—not too hot or too cold, although cooler temperatures are generally more conducive to sleep. Also, make sure your room is as dark as possible.

o   Avoid exercising within three hours of bedtime and eating large meals close to bedtime because this can keep you awake. It is also a good idea to avoid consuming caffeine past noon and drinking alcohol close to bedtime.

☐ **Be social.** This doesn't mean that you need to be the most amusing person in the room. It does mean getting together with people, accepting invitations, answering the phone, responding to texts and emails, and being active in the community.

☐ **Minimize distractions and increase focus.** Being able to concentrate on a task and do it well is a major promoter of brain health. Try to minimize the distracters around you in order to settle down to complete a task with your full attention.

☐ **Protect your hearing.** Hearing loss can contribute to the loss of grey matter in the brain and increase the risk of cognitive impairment. Be careful of sustained loud noises in close proximity to your ears.

☐ **Challenge your mind.** The phrase "use it or lose it" definitely applies here. One great way to promote brain health is through giving your brain a workout. You can do this in several ways:

o Do crossword puzzles, Sudoku, and other games, including online brain games such as those at Lumosity or Happy Neuron.

o Learn new skills (a new language, a musical instrument, or a new hobby).

o Reduce dependence on devices and other mental crutches. For example, without relying on GPS, take a different route to work or walk around an unfamiliar part of the city (that's safe, of course). If you're feeling really ambitious, navigate a new city without GPS.

o Read a variety of books and articles on topics of interest to you.

o   Take classes to improve your knowledge or just for fun.

Don't:

☐   **Overeat**. Especially don't consume too much sugar and processed snack food. If you follow a diet like MIND, then you won't be in danger of overloading on sugar and processed food that can harm cognitive function. Trans fats, which are a major part of junk food, harden cell membranes, slowing brain function. Too much sugar in your blood can cause brain matter to atrophy or shrink and impede the formation of necessary functional connections in the brain. (Too little blood sugar can also be a problem, which is why a well-balanced, adequate diet is so essential.) Let's break this down:

o   According to the American Heart Association, men should consume no more than 9 teaspoons of sugar daily. That's 36 grams. Women should consume no more than 6 teaspoons daily, or 25 grams. According to the World Health Organization (WHO), sugar should be no more than 10% of an adult's diet, and ideally less than 5%.

o   One 12-ounce can of Coca-Cola contains 39 grams of sugar. You can easily see that, even for men, one can of Coke is the entire day's sugar allotment.

o   Diet Coke and Coke Zero have no calories and no sugar, but what they do have is nonnutritive sweeteners. Unlike natural sugars, these sweeteners are not converted by the body into energy or fat. So, they don't add calories, but they have no nutritional benefit either. They also may have negative long-term effects, such as increasing the risk of developing type 2 diabetes and other types of metabolic dysregulation. Diet soft drinks don't give your body anything it can use, and that can cause problems.

o It's not just sugar that's the enemy, as you can see. It's any food or drink that has no or negative nutritional value. That describes junk food in general, which tends to be high in trans fats and phosphorus and low in anything else that your body needs and can use. Junk food has little to no fiber and generally none of the essential phytonutrients that fruits and vegetables provide. It raises LDL cholesterol and increases the risk of high blood pressure, obesity, and acne.

o Junk food is also addictive, sometimes by design because of the artificial sweeteners and sometimes because junk food depresses the pleasure response to food in the brain, which causes overeating to compensate.

o It's best to cut out junk food from your diet. You don't need it. Soft drinks are the same. Get your daily allotment of sugar from things like fruits and vegetables instead, foods that produce genuine pleasure to eat because they taste good, don't provoke overeating, and provide your body with fiber and a rich array of essential nutrients.

☐ **Multitask.** Research shows that—contrary to popular belief—multitasking is not doing several things at once; rather, it is switching among tasks constantly. Focused, concentrated action is good for the brain. Unfocused jumping around from task to task disrupts focus and weakens brain function.

- [ ] **Drink too much alcohol.** Diets like the Mediterranean diet do call for a moderate amount of wine consumption (that is, if you drink alcohol at all), but drinking to excess is not healthy for your brain, your liver, or the rest of your body. For example, chronic drinking to excess can cause emotional disturbances such as depression and anxiety. It can also cause severe brain damage, leading to conditions such as Wernicke-Korsakoff syndrome (WKS), which involves amnesia, extreme confusion, and visual disturbances.

- [ ] **Smoke.** Cigarette tobacco contains an addictive substance, nicotine. Nicotine produces a stimulant effect, releasing adrenaline in the body, and it activates the reward circuits in the brain. It also increases the level of dopamine, a chemical messenger that motivates behaviors that will produce more of the reward-stimulating effect. (Electronic cigarettes, used in what is commonly called "vaping," also contain nicotine and produce this addictive effect on the brain.) This means you'll keep smoking, which produces a broad range of ill effects that can cause symptoms such as irritability, loss of sleep, decreased attention span, and increased appetite if you try to quit. Smoking also causes lung issues that decrease oxygen intake and, consequently, have detrimental effects on the brain. In short, none of the effects of smoking are conducive to long-term brain health.

- [ ] **Sit for prolonged periods of time without a break.** If you get up every once in a while throughout the day to move around, you increase your energy and the blood flow to your brain— which can perk you up and keep your brain working at a higher level.

☐ **Spend too much time on one thing,** such as too much time watching TV or staring at social media. Engage your mind. It's not that screen time is necessarily bad, but being engaged and using your brain is better than just scrolling through a celebrity's Instagram feed.

Conclusion

Alzheimer's disease and dementia are often very difficult diseases to confront, both for those who have the ailment and their loved ones. As more research is conducted on these diseases, helpful information is released to the public. Research on nutritional changes is a growing and increasingly popular field, especially as more data is collected regarding the many positive benefits of a healthy diet. Whether you have a family history of Alzheimer's disease or dementia, are at risk for the disease, or have a loved one who is suffering, the nutritional changes discussed here could be very helpful. Many of these dietary modifications decrease a person's risk factors for developing Alzheimer's disease or dementia or slow progression of the disease. In addition, most of the health guidelines discussed in this book not only benefit brain health but overall health as well..

About the Authors

Laura Town

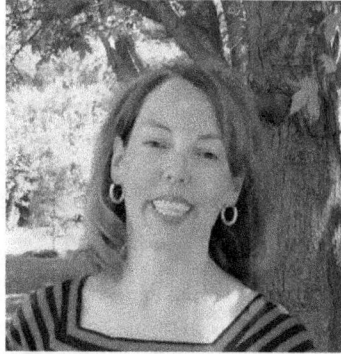

Laura Town has authored numerous publications of special interest to the aging population. She has written for the American Medical Writers Association, and her work has been published by the American Society of Journalists and Authors. As an editor and instructional designer, Laura has worked with Pearson Education, WebMD, California State University, National PACE Association, and the University of Pennsylvania to create both on-ground and online courses and texts. She is the past president of the Indiana chapter of the American Medical Writers Association. Laura's book *Dementia, Alzheimer's Disease Stages, Treatments, and Other Medical Considerations* is one of Book Authority's top ten best-selling print books about dementia and top 100 best audiobooks about dementia of all time. In her spare time, Laura writes creatively. Her novel on Victoria Woodhull (under the pseudonym Eva Flynn) won the 2015 gold medal and her play *A Touch* of *Glory* about the 1955 Crispus Attucks team was supported by the Lilly Foundation.

Karen Hoffman

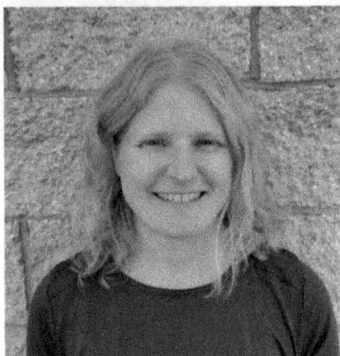

Karen Hoffman received her Ph.D. in Pharmacology from the Department of Pharmacology and Experimental Neurosciences at the University of Nebraska Medical Center in Omaha, NE, where she was the recipient of an American Heart Association fellowship and several regional and national awards for her research on G protein-coupled receptor signaling in airways. She then pursued post-doctoral research projects at the University of North Carolina-Chapel Hill and the University of Kansas Medical Center, again receiving fellowships from the PhRMA Foundation and the American Heart Association, respectively. She has published research in the American Journal of Pathology, Journal of Biological Chemistry, and Journal of Pharmacology and Experimental Therapeutics. In 2012, Karen joined the editorial staff at WilliamsTown Communications, an editing firm that specializes in educational products for undergraduate- and graduate-level students. At WTC, Karen specializes in producing educational products related to the sciences and healthcare. In addition, Karen is board-certified for editing life sciences (BELS-certified).

A Note from the Authors

Thank you for purchasing our book! Worldwide, nearly 50 million people suffer from Alzheimer's disease or other forms of dementia, and that number is expected to increase significantly within the next 15 years. In the United States, more than 5 million people have Alzheimer's disease, and that is expected to nearly triple by the year 2050.

Despite these large numbers, you may feel alone. I (Laura) know that when I started caring for my father, who had early-onset Alzheimer's disease, I felt alone. Although my father has passed away, I am haunted by what he suffered and how difficult it was to care for him. However, now I know that there are people, resources, and organizations that can help others going through this same struggle.

One major concern of caregivers is knowing how to provide adequate nutrition for their loved one. We hope that the information in the *Alzheimer's Roadmap* series will ease some of your stress. The information provided in this book not only provides guidelines on what types of foods will most benefit your loved one's cognitive function but also how to prepare those foods so your loved one can consume them easily and safely. In addition, we have included resources at the end of this book to provide additional information to help you through this process.

If you have any questions, please reach out to Laura via LinkedIn: https://www.linkedin.com/in/lauratown. We would appreciate it if you would take the time to review our book on Amazon, as our book's visibility on Amazon depends on reviews.

More Titles from Laura Town and Karen Hoffman

Alzheimer's Roadmap series:

Long-Term Care Insurance, Power of Attorney, Wealth Management, and Other First Steps

Dementia, Alzheimer's Disease Stages, Treatment Options, and Other Medical Considerations

Advance Directives, Durable Power of Attorney, Wills, and Other Legal Considerations

Coping with Dementia

Enhancing Activities of Daily Living

Home Safety Checklist Guide and Caregiver Resources for Medication Safety, Driving, and Wandering

Paying for Healthcare and Other Financial Considerations

Home Care, Long-term Care, Memory Care Units, and Other Living Arrangements

Caregiver Resources: From Independence to a Memory Care Unit

Nutrition for Brain Health: Fighting Dementia

Final Steps: End of Life Care for Dementia

Other titles:

How to Save Money on Healthcare

Where Should Mom Live?

Protect Yourself & Your Family

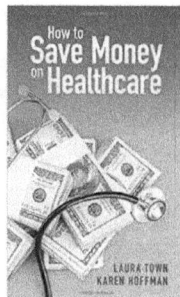

Advance Directives, Durable Power of Attorney, Wills, and Other Legal Considerations provides answers to the following questions and more:

- **How do I get a handle on my finances?** Find out what you need in order to pass on your financial information to others.
- **How do I transfer wealth to my loved ones?** Create a plan for transferring wealth, setting up joint ownership of accounts, and preparing for the tax implications of transfer.
- **What types of insurance should I have?** Walk through the various types of insurance policies, including long-term care insurance, disability insurance, and life insurance.
- **What legal documents for finances and healthcare do I need?** Explore durable powers of attorney for finances and healthcare, a last will and testament, a living trust, a living will, and advance directives.
- **Is there an audio version of this book?** Yes, there is. You can find it at: https://amzn.to/2tAS91c

Resources

Alzheimer's Association
225 N. Michigan Ave., Fl. 17
Chicago, IL 60601-7633
Phone: 800-272-3900
Website: http://www.alz.org

Alzheimer's Foundation of America
322 Eighth Ave., 16th fl.
New York, NY 10001
Phone: 866-232-8484
Email: info@alzfdn.org
Website: www.alzfdn.org

MyPlate
Website: https://www.myplate.gov
MyPlate is a good resource for creating a customized daily
food plan.

Alzheimer's Roadmap series:

*Long-Term Care Insurance, Power of Attorney, Wealth
Management, and Other First Steps*

*Dementia, Alzheimer's Disease Stages, Treatment Options, and
Other Medical Considerations*

*Advance Directives, Durable Power of Attorney, Wills, and Other
Legal Considerations*

Coping with Dementia

Enhancing Activities of Daily Living

Home Safety Checklist Guide and Caregiver Resources for

Medication Safety, Driving, and Wandering

Paying for Healthcare and Other Financial Considerations

Home Care, Long-term Care, Memory Care Units, and Other Living Arrangements

Caregiver Resources: From Independence to a Memory Care Unit

Nutrition for Brain Health: Fighting Dementia

Final Steps: End of Life Care for Dementia

Reference List

Action for Happiness (n.d.). Set your goals and make them happen. Retrieved from https://www.actionforhappiness.org/take-action/set-your-goals-and-make-them-happen

Alzheimer's Association. (2016). Retrieved from http://www.alz.org/

Alzheimer's Association. (2020). 2020 Alzheimer's disease facts and figures. Retrieved from https://www.alz.org/media/Documents/alzheimers-facts-and-figures.pdf

Alzheimer's Association. (2021). Causes and risk factors for Alzheimer's disease. Retrieved from https://www.alz.org/alzheimers-dementia/what-is-alzheimers/causes-and-risk-factors

Alzheimer's Association. (2024). 2024 Alzheimer's disease facts and figures. *Alzheimer's & Dementia, 20*(5), 3708–3821. https://doi.org/10.1002/alz.13809

Alzheimer's Society. (n.d.). *Obesity and dementia risk*. Retrieved July 2024 from https://www.alzheimers.org.uk/about-dementia/managing-the-risk-of-dementia/reduce-your-risk-of-dementia/obesity

Alzheimer's Society. (2021). Eating and drinking. Retrieved from http://www.alzheimers.org.uk/site/scripts/documents_info.php?documentID=149

American Dental Association. (n.d.). *Cannabis: Oral health effects*. https://www.ada.org/en/resources/ada-library/oral-health-topics/cannabis-oral-health-effects

American Heart Association. (2021). Saturated Fats. Retrieved from http://www.heart.org/HEARTORG/GettingHealthy/NutritionCenter/HealthyEating/Saturated-Fats_UCM_301110_Article.jsp

American Heart Association Newsroom. (2024, March 18). *8-hour time-restricted eating linked to a 91% higher risk of cardiovascular death*. American Heart Association. https://newsroom.heart.org/news/8-hour-time-restricted-eating-linked-to-a-91-higher-risk-of-cardiovascular-death

American Stroke Association. (2021). About stroke. Retrieved from https://www.stroke.org/en/about-stroke

Arora, M., ElSayed, A., Beger, B., Naidoo, P., Shilton, T., Jain, N., Armstrong-Walenczak, K., Mwangi, J., Wang, Y., Eiselé, J. L., Pinto, F. J., & Champagne, B. M. (2022). The impact of alcohol consumption on cardiovascular health: Myths and measures. *Global Heart, 17*(1), 45. https://doi.org/10.5334/gh.1132

Arora, S., Santiago, J. A., Bernstein, M., & Potashkin, J. A. (2023). Diet and lifestyle impact the development and progression of Alzheimer's dementia. *Frontiers in Nutrition, 10*, 1213223. https://doi.org/10.3389/fnut.2023.1213223

Baillie, K. U. (2022, March 4). *One alcoholic drink a day linked with reduced brain size.* University of Pennsylvania, Penn Today. https://penntoday.upenn.edu/news/one-alcoholic-drink-day-linked-reduced-brain-size

Being Patient. (2018). Can you fight Alzheimer's with a cup of coffee? Retrieved from https://www.beingpatient.com/coffee-prevent-alzheimers/

Biddinger, K. J., Emdin, C. A., Haas, M. E., Wang, M., Hindy, G., Ellinor, P. T., Kathiresan, S., Khera, A. V., & Aragam, K. G. (2022). Association of habitual alcohol intake with risk of cardiovascular disease. *JAMA Network Open, 5*(3), e223849-e223849.

Blaha, M. J. (2021). 5 vaping facts you need to know. *Johns Hopkins Medicine.* Retrieved from https://www.hopkinsmedicine.org/health/wellness-and-prevention/5-truths-you-need-to-know-about-vaping

Chen, J. T., Tsai, S., Chen, M. H., Pitiphat, W., Matangkasombut, O., Chiou, J. M., Han, M. L., Chen, J. H., & Chen, Y. C. (2024). Association between oral health and cognitive impairment in older adults: Insights from a six-year prospective cohort study. *Journal of Dentistry, 147*, Article 105088. https://doi.org/10.1016/j.jdent.2024.105088

Children's Hospital of Philadelphia. (2022, December 21). *Food as medicine: Prebiotic foods.* https://www.chop.edu/health-resources/food-medicine-prebiotic-foods

Cleveland Clinic. (n.d.). *Oral hygiene.* Retrieved July 2024 from https://my.clevelandclinic.org/health/treatments/16914-oral-hygiene

Cleveland Clinic. (2019). Eating and nutritional challenges in patients with Alzheimer's disease: Tips for caregivers. Retrieved from http://my.clevelandclinic.org/health/articles/9597-eating-and-nutritional-challenges-in-patients-with-alzheimers-disease-tips-for-caregivers

Cleveland Clinic. (2020). Fad diets. Retrieved from https://my.clevelandclinic.org/health/articles/9476-fad-diets

Cleveland Clinic. (2020). 6 pillars of brain health. Retrieved from https://healthybrains.org/pillars/

CocaCola Co. (2021). How much sugar in Coke is there? Retrieved from https://www.coca-colacompany.com/faqs/how-much-sugar-is-in-coca-cola

ConsumerFinance.gov. (2018). Setting SMART goals. Retrieved from https://files.consumerfinance.gov/f/documents/cfpb_your-money-your-goals_SMART-goals_tool_2018-11.pdf

Crichton-Stuart, C. (2020). What are the benefits of eating healthy? *Medical News Today*. Retrieved from https://www.medicalnewstoday.com/articles/322268#weight-loss

Daviet, R., Aydogan, G., Jagannathan, K., Spilka, N., Koellinger, P. D., Kranzler, H. R., Nave, G., & Wetherill, R. R. (2022). Associations between alcohol consumption and gray and white matter volumes in the UK Biobank. *Nature Communications, 13,* Article 1175. https://doi.org/10.1038/s41467-022-28735-5

Davis, J. C., Bryan, S., Marra, C. A., Sharma, D., Chan, A., Beattie, B. L., Graf, P., & Liu-Amrose, T. (2013). An economic evaluation of resistance training and aerobic training versus balance and toning exercises in older adults with mild cognitive impairment. PLoS One, 8(5), e63031.

De la Rosa, A., Olaso-Gonzalez, G., Arc-Chagnaud, C., Millan, F., Salvador-Pascual, A., Garcia-Lucerga, C., Blasco-Lafarga, C., Garcia-Dominquez, E., Carretero, A., Correas, A., Vina, J., Gomez-Cabrera, M.C.. (2020). Physical exercise in the prevention and treatment of Alzheimer's disease. *Journal of Sport and Health Science.* 9(5), 394-404. Retrieved from https://www.sciencedirect.com/science/article/pii/S2095254620300119

DiGiulio, S. (2021). 7 do's and don'ts for a better-working brain. *Men's Journal.* Retrieved from https://www.mensjournal.com/food-drink/seven-dos-and-donts-for-a-better-working-brain/

Downey, M. (2014, August). How green tea protects against Alzheimer's disease. *Life Extension Magazine.* Retrieved in February 2020 from http://www.lef.org/Magazine/2014/8/How-Green-Tea-Protects-Against-Alzheimers-Disease/Page-01

Ducharme, J. (2023, January 19). Is there really no safe amount of drinking? *TIME.* https://time.com/6248439/no-safe-amount-of-alcohol/

Edwards, S. (2020). Sugar and the brain. *Harvard Medical School.* Retrieved in February 2020 from https://neuro.hms.harvard.edu/harvard-mahoney-neuroscience-institute/brain-newsletter/and-brain-series/sugar-and-brain

Ellouze, I., Sheffler, J., Nagpal, R., & Arjmandi, B. (2023). Dietary patterns and Alzheimer's disease: An updated review linking nutrition to neuroscience. *Nutrients, 15*(14), 3204. https://doi.org/10.3390/nu15143204

Ensle, K. (2013) How to quickly spot a fad diet. Retrieved from https://njaes.rutgers.edu/sshw/message/message.php?p=Health&m=233

Fitzgerald Dentistry. (2023, January 10). *Tobacco use and oral health: Avoid for better tomorrow.* https://www.fitzgeralddentistry.com/blog/tobacco-use-oral-health-cancer/

Food and Drug Administration. (2020). Selecting and serving fresh and frozen seafood safely. Retrieved from http://www.fda.gov/food/buy-store-serve-safe-food/selecting-and-serving-fresh-and-frozen-seafood-safely

Food for the Brain. (2021). Positive action on Alzheimer's. Retrieved from http://www.foodforthebrain.org/campaigns/alzheimers/

Galvin, J. (2019). Lewy body dementia. *Practical Neurology.* Retrieved from https://practicalneurology.com/articles/2019-june/lewy-body-dementia-1

Grant, M. (n.d.). Brain tips: 27 things you can do to care for your brain.

Overcoming Pain. Retrieved from https://overcomingpain.com/self-help/brain-tips-27-things-you-can-do-to-care-for-your-brain/

Greenfield, N. (2015). The smart seafood buying guide. Retrieved from https://www.nrdc.org/stories/smart-seafood-buying-guide.

Haiken, M. (2013, June 30). Green tea may prevent Alzheimer's disease, says four new studies. *Forbes.* Retrieved from http://www.forbes.com/sites/melaniehaiken/2013/06/30/green-tea-may-prevent-alzheimers-say-four-new-studies/

Harvard Health Publishing. (2019). By the way, doctor: What's the right amount of vitamin C for me? Retrieved in February 2020 from https://www.health.harvard.edu/staying-healthy/whats-the-right-amount-of-vitamin-c-for-me

Harvard Publishing Staff. (2022, August 9). Ketogenic diet: Is the ultimate low-carb diet good for you? *Harvard Health.* https://www.health.harvard.edu/blog/ketogenic-diet-is-the-ultimate-low-carb-diet-good-for-you-2017072712089

Harvard School of Public Health. (2021). Fish: Friend or foe? Retrieved from http://www.hsph.harvard.edu/nutritionsource/fish/

Healthline. (2020). The benefits of healthy habits. Retrieved in February 2020 from https://www.healthline.com/health/5-benefits-healthy-habits

Healthy Women. (2017, July 26). Do's and don'ts for brain health. *Brain Health.* Retrieved from https://www.healthywomen.org/content/article/dos-and-donts-brain-health

Heston, M. B., Hanslik, K. L., Zarbock, K. R., Harding, S. J., Davenport-Sis, N. J., Kerby, R. L., Chin, N., Sun, Y., Hoeft, A., Deming, Y., Vogt, N. M., Betthauser, T. J., Johnson, S. C., Asthana, S., Kollmorgen, G., Suridjan, I., Wild, N., Zetterberg, H., Blennow, K.,...Ulland, T. K. (2023). Gut inflammation associated with age and Alzheimer's disease pathology: A human cohort study. *Scientific Reports, 13,* Article 18924. https://doi.org/10.1038/s41598-023-45929-z

HHS.gov. (n.d.). Importance of Good Nutrition. Retrieved in February 2020 from https://www.hhs.gov/fitness/eat-healthy/importance-of-good-nutrition/index.html

Hu, N., Yu, J., Wang, Y., Sun, L., & Tan, L. (2013). Nutrition and the risk of Alzheimer's disease. *BioMed Research International*, 2013 (5248204), 1-12.

Jicha, G., & Swaminathan, A. (2014). Nutrition and prevention of Alzheimer's dementia. *Frontiers in Aging Neuroscience*, 6(282), 1-25.

Kim, K. Y., Ha, J., Lee, J. Y., & Kim, E. (2023). Weight loss and risk of dementia in individuals with versus without obesity. *Alzheimer's & Dementia, 19*(12), 5471–5481. https://doi.org/10.1002/alz.13155

Lama, S. (2020). Can you juice your vegetables instead of eating them? *Livestrong*. Retrieved from http://www.livestrong.com/article/251138-benefits-of-juicing-vs-eating-your-vegetables/

Leite, S. O., Batista, G. F., Magalhães, V. B., Oliveira, A. K. A., & Dias, K. S. P. A. (2024). Interrelation between periodontal and Alzheimer's disease: Integrative review. *Interconnections of Knowledge: Multidisciplinary Approaches, 45*, 733–744. https://doi.org/10.56238/sevened2024.010-045

Li, J., Liu, C., Ang, T. F. A., & Au, R. (2023). BMI decline patterns and relation to dementia risk across four decades of follow-up in the Framingham Study. *Alzheimer's & Dementia, 19*(6), 2520–2527. https://doi.org/10.1002/alz.12839

Liang, Y., Liu, C., Cheng, M., Geng, L., Li, J., Du, W., Song, M., Chen, N., Yeleen, T. A. N., Song, L., Wang, X., Han, Y., & Sheng, C. (2024). The link between gut microbiome and Alzheimer's disease: From the perspective of new revised criteria for diagnosis and staging of Alzheimer's disease. *Alzheimer's & Dementia*. Advance online publication. https://doi.org/10.1002/alz.14057

Lin, J., Pathak, J. L., Shen, Y., Mashrah, M. A., Zhong, X., Chen, J., Li, Z., Xia, J., Liang, Y., & Zeng, Y. (2024). Association between periodontitis and mild cognitive impairment: A systematic review and meta-analysis. *Dementia and Geriatric Cognitive Disorders, 53*(1), 37–46. https://doi.org/10.1159/000535776

Liu, X., Wang, Y., Dhana, K., Agarwal, P., Cherian, L. J., Bennett, D. A., Schneider, J. A., & Aggarwal, N. T. (2021). Plant-based dietary patterns and cognitive function in US adults: A prospective evaluation. *Alzheimer's & Dementia, 17*(Suppl 10), e054349. https://doi.org/10.1002/alz.054349

Mayo Clinic. (n.d.). How to make the keto diet healthy. Retrieved July 2024 from https://diet.mayoclinic.org/us/blog/2022/how-to-make-the-keto-diet-healthy/

Mayo Clinic. (2019). Improve brain health with the MIND diet. Retrieved from https://www.mayoclinic.org/healthy-lifestyle/nutrition-and-healthy-eating/in-depth/improve-brain-health-with-the-mind-diet/art-20454746

Mayo Clinic. (2020). Health lifestyle: Stress management. Retrieved from https://www.mayoclinic.org/healthy-lifestyle/stress-management/in-depth/stress-relief/art-20044476

Mayo Clinic. (2020). Water: How much should you drink every day? Retrieved from https://www.mayoclinic.org/healthy-lifestyle/nutrition-and-healthy-eating/in-depth/water/art-20044256

McMorrow, L., Ludbrook, A., Macdiarmid, J., and Olajide, D. (2016). Perceived barriers towards healthy eating and their association with fruit and vegetable consumption. *Journal of Public Health*, 39(2), 3300-338. Retrieved from https://academic.oup.com/jpubhealth/article/39/2/330/3002965

MedlinePlus. (2021). Retrieved from http://www.nlm.nih.gov/medlineplus/

Menon, S. (2016). Mercury guide. Retrieved from https://www.nrdc.org/stories/mercury-guide.

MyPlate. (n.d.). MyPlate Plan. Retrieved from https://www.myplate.gov/myplate-plan

National Center for Health Statistics. (n.d.). *Glossary—Alcohol.* U.S. Department of Health & Human Services, Centers for Disease Control and Prevention. Retrieved July 2024 from https://www.cdc.gov/nchs/nhis/alcohol/alcohol_glossary.htm

National Institute of Dental and Craniofacial Research. (n.d.). *Oral hygiene.* U.S. Department of Health and Human Services, National Institutes of Health. Retrieved July 2024 from https://www.nidcr.nih.gov/health-info/oral-hygiene

National Institute on Aging. (2016). A good night's sleep. Retrieved from https://www.nia.nih.gov/health/good-nights-sleep

National Institute on Aging. (2023, June 12). *Beyond the brain: The gut microbiome and Alzheimer's disease.* U.S. Department of Health & Human Services, National Institutes of Health. https://www.nia.nih.gov/news/beyond-brain-gut-microbiome-and-alzheimers-disease

National Institute on Drug Abuse. (2020). Cigarettes and other tobacco products. *DrugFacts.* Retrieved from https://www.drugabuse.gov/publications/drugfacts/cigarettes-other-tobacco-products

National Institutes of Health Office of Dietary Supplements. (2020). Vitamin K. Retrieved from https://ods.od.nih.gov/factsheets/VitaminK-HealthProfessional/

National Institutes of Health Office of Dietary Supplements. (2021). Vitamin D. Retrieved from https://ods.od.nih.gov/factsheets/VitaminD-Consumer/

Norman, A. (2024, July 2). *Leaky gut diet: What to eat and sample meals.* Verywell Health. https://www.verywellhealth.com/leaky-gut-diet-4773680

NSW Health. (2021, September 17). *Healthy habits for a healthy mouth.* NSW Government. https://www.health.nsw.gov.au/oralhealth/prevention/Pages/healthy-habits.aspx

NutritionFacts.org. (n.d.). Junk food. Retrieved from https://nutritionfacts.org/topics/junk-food/

Pike, A. (2019). What is the MIND diet? Retrieved from https://foodinsight.org/what-is-the-mind-diet/

Precker, M. (2020, August 26). *Need another reason not to vape? Your oral health is at risk.* American Heart Association News. https://www.heart.org/en/news/2020/08/26/need-another-reason-not-to-vape-your-oral-health-is-at-risk

Raman, R. (2013, March 17). *The leaky gut diet plan: What to eat, what to avoid.* https://www.healthline.com/nutrition/leaky-gut-diet

Reynolds, G. (2014). Can exercise reduce Alzheimer's risk? *The New York Times.* Retrieved from

http://well.blogs.nytimes.com/2014/07/02/can-exercise-reduce-
alzheimers-risk/?_r=0

Ries, J. (2023, May 12). *Can Ozempic and other GLP-1 drugs reduce your
dementia disease risk?* Healthline. https://www.healthline.com/health-
news/can-ozempic-and-other-glp-1-drugs-reduce-alzheimers-disease-
risk

Robinson, L., Smith, M., & Segal, R. (2020). Stress management.
HelpGuide. Retrieved from
https://www.helpguide.org/articles/stress/stress-management.htm

Robson, D. (2015). Dos and don'ts to preserve your brainpower. *BBC
Future.* Retrieved from https://www.bbc.com/future/article/20150828-
dos-and-donts-to-preserve-your-brainpower

Shabir, O. (2019, February 26). *Alzheimer's disease and the microbiome.*
News-Medical.net. https://www.news-medical.net/health/Alzheimers-
Disease-and-the-Microbiome.aspx

Sifferlin, A. (2012, July 16). Mind your reps: Exercise, especially weight
lifting, helps keep the brain sharp. *Time.* Retrieved from
http://healthland.time.com/2012/07/16/mind-those-reps-exercise-
especially-weight-lifting-helps-keep-your-brain-sharp/

Signature Smile Family Dentistry & Orthodontics. (n.d.). 10 *great ways to
take care of your teeth.* Retrieved July 2024 from
https://signaturesmiledfw.com/10-great-ways-to-take-care-of-your-
teeth/

Singh-Manoux, A., Dugravot, A., Shipley, M., Brunner, E. J., Elbaz, A.,
Sabia, S., & Kivimaki, M. (2018). Obesity trajectories and risk of
dementia: 28 years of follow-up in the Whitehall II Study. *Alzheimer's &
Dementia, 14*(2), 178–186. https://doi.org/10.1016/j.jalz.2017.06.2637

Sizar, O., Khare, S., Goyal, A., Bansal, P., Givler, A. (2020). Vitamin D.
Deficiency. *NCBI Bookshelf.* Retrieved from
https://www.ncbi.nih.gov/books/NBK532266/

Smith, M., Robinson, L., & Segal, J. (2020). Alzheimer's and dementia:
Preventing Alzheimer's disease and dementia. Retrieved from
http://www.helpguide.org/articles/alzheimers-dementia-
aging/preventing-alzheimers-disease.htm

Southwick, C. (2024, February 27). *10 best and worst foods for leaky gut, according to dietitians*. Eating Well. https://www.eatingwell.com/leaky-gut-diet-8600895

Spritzler, F. (2018). 10 Magnesium-rich foods that are super healthy. Retrieved from https://www.healthline.com/nutrition/10-foods-high-in-magnesium#section3

Stibich, M. (2020). 9 great brain games and brain training websites. Retrieved from https://www.verywellmind.com/top-websites-and-games-for-brain-exercise-2224140

University of California. (n.d.). SMART goals: A how to guide. Retrieved from https://www.ucop.edu/local-human-resources/_files/performance-appraisal/How%20to%20write%20SMART%20Goals%20v2.pdf

University of California San Francisco. (n.d.). How much is too much? The growing concern over too much added sugar in our diets. *SugarScience*. Retrieved from https://sugarscience.ucsf.edu/the-growing-concern-of-overconsumption.html#.XjhypndFyUk

University of California San Francisco Well Institute for Neurosciences. (n.d.). The Mediterranean diet pyramid. Retrieved from https://memory.ucsf.edu/sites/memory.ucsf.edu/files/Mediterranean DietHandout.pdf

University of Illinois Chicago College of Dentistry. (2022, March 23). *Cannabis and its impact on oral health*. https://dentistry.uic.edu/news-stories/cannabis-and-its-impact-on-oral-health/

U.S. News and World Report. (2021). Best diets overall. Retrieved from https://health.usnews.com/best-diet/best-diets-overall

U.S. News and World Report. (2021). What is MIND diet? Retrieved from https://health.usnews.com/best-diet/mind-diet

Victoria State Government BetterHealth Channel. (2020). Weight loss and fad diets. Retrieved from https://www.betterhealth.vic.gov.au/health/healthyliving/weight-loss-and-fad-diets

World Health Organization. (2020). Dementia. Retrieved from https://www.who.int/news-room/fact-sheets/detail/dementia

World Health Organization. (2023, January 4). *No level of alcohol consumption is safe for our health* [News release]. https://www.who.int/europe/news/item/04-01-2023-no-level-of-alcohol-consumption-is-safe-for-our-health

Zhang, E. (2018, June 3). Diet drinks may seem like a good idea, but their effects may surprise you. *Washington Post*. Retrieved from https://www.washingtonpost.com/national/health-science/diet-drinks-may-seem-like-a-good-idea-but-their-effects-may-surprise-you/2018/06/01/85859710-5d06-11e8-a4a4-c070ef53f315_story.html

Art Credits

1. U.S. Department of Health and Human Services
2. Dragon Images
3. SpeedKingz
4. NataliTerr
5. kurhan
6. Mykola Komarovskyy
7. Robyn Mackenzie
8. margouillat photo
9. alexapro9500
10. Jacek Chabraszewski
11. Laura Town
12. Karen Hoffman

Continue reading to see a selection from another Omega Press title, available now on Amazon.

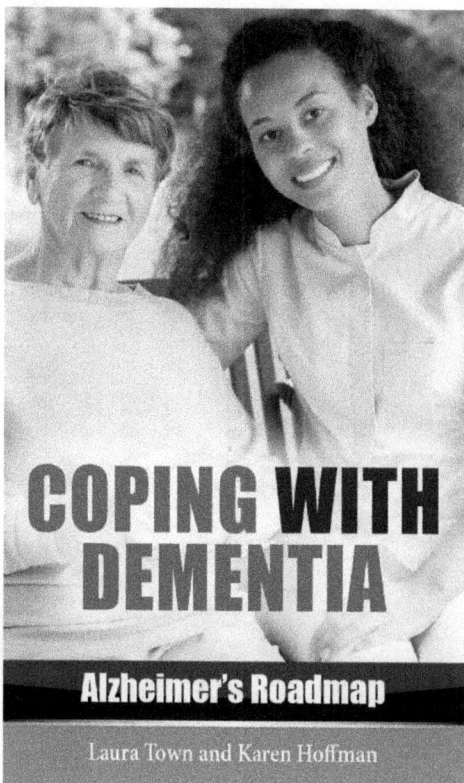

COPING WITH DEMENTIA

Alzheimer's Roadmap

Laura Town and Karen Hoffman

Coping with Dementia

People, whether they be friends or strangers, will be sympathetic when you tell them that a loved one has dementia. Not knowing how to respond, people will try to find something positive to say about your tragedy—and dementia is tragic. The one comment that bothered me (Laura) the most, although the intention behind it was good, was that at least my father "doesn't know what's happening to him." This is completely false. My dad, in the early and even in the mid stages, knew what was happening. Yes, he couldn't articulate it all the time. Yes, he could not go into detail about the functions of the brain or give a scientific explanation of what was happening. But he knew that he could no longer complete simple tasks. He cried when he could no longer drive. He was enraged when he could not remember the names of his relatives. And he sank into a deep depression when he had to start wearing adult diapers. Even in the late stages when dad was living in a locked dementia unit and before he became nonverbal, my father pointed to adults rocking baby dolls and said to me that he wished he wasn't one of "those people."

Dad's doctor told me that if you've seen one case of Alzheimer's disease, it just means that you've seen one case of Alzheimer's disease, meaning that all cases are different. Perhaps some people slide straight from complete cognition to the late stages of Alzheimer's disease and truly do not have any frustration while being in the throes of the disease, but I have never heard of this.

So people with dementia do know, on a fundamental level, what is happening. That doesn't mean that they know it every day, or even every hour, or become obsessed with their declining health. Dad still had happy moments. He still enjoyed taking walks, listening to music, seeing his grandsons, and eating cupcakes. As long as he was able, I still took him out to restaurants for lunch and dinner or brought him to my house. And although he wasn't particularly religious, he enjoyed visits with the ministers and volunteers who came and read the Bible to him. The challenge is to find what your loved one enjoys and then try to incorporate the enjoyment of it into as many moments of their life as you are able. If you are the one suffering from dementia, then think about what gives you pleasure and find a way to do those things as often as you are able.

When your loved one is diagnosed with Alzheimer's disease or another type of dementia, the emotional effect on the whole family is tremendous. As much as possible, the person with dementia has to come to terms with living with a terminal degenerative disease. They must reckon with a failing memory as well as an increasing reliance on others while also dealing with a society that may feel they have lost their value. Once they enter middle- and later-stage dementia, the disease will begin to affect emotional responses as well as the ability to communicate.

Caregivers, family, and friends of the person with dementia must also process powerful emotions about the news. If your parent, spouse, or other loved one is diagnosed with dementia, you might experience grief over your loved one's loss of memory as well as confusion and stress over practical medical, legal, and financial issues. Your family will likely face some major challenges as you collectively adapt to meet the new needs of the person with dementia. Most significantly, the day-to-day stress of caregiving can take a profound toll on your physical and mental well-being. Being a caregiver affects all parts of your life—personal, professional, and financial—and you may feel that you don't have more than a few minutes to yourself each day. This daily stress can continue for years—sometimes a decade or longer—with serious health implications for you and your family. Studies have found that caregivers' own health problems can be caused or exacerbated by the constant stress of providing care. Studies have also shown that stressed caregivers effectively age faster than people without chronic caregiving responsibilities. According to an American Association of Retired Persons (AARP) report from 2015, 34.2 million Americans provided unpaid care to an adult age 50 or older in the prior 12 months. According to the same report, caregivers spend an average of 24.4 hours a week providing care, with nearly a quarter spending 41 hours or more on care each week, and those caring for a spouse or partner spending 44.6 hours a week. That's an enormous time investment that leaves significantly less time for paid employment and leisure activities. It's easy to see from this how easily caregiving can become all-consuming for the people who provide it.

This book examines the emotional fallout of dementia, and specifically how people with the disease, their caregivers, and their non-caregiver family and friends can cope with that fallout. You'll read about the stages of the disease and how to cope with the common changes at each step. You'll also read about problems that often accompany a terminal chronic illness such as Alzheimer's disease—depression, anxiety, anger, guilt, sleep disturbances, and suicide risk—and how to respond healthily to each of these problems. You'll also get tips and advice for how to support others over the course of dementia:

the loved one with the disease, other caregivers, and other family and friends. Although there are different types of dementia including Alzheimer's disease, our checklists should be applicable regardless of the specific diagnosis, and so "dementia" is the term used throughout this book for Alzheimer's disease and other types.

Emotional Considerations for the Individual with Dementia

Dementia destroys the cognitive function of the individual with the disease. Its effects are catastrophic. The reality is that if you have dementia, you will not only lose the ability to think and remember clearly. You will experience extreme behavioral and emotional changes as the disease progresses, will no longer recognize family members or close friends, and may even develop irrational fears and paranoias. Everyone experiences a loss of function and independence as they age. This is often an emotional struggle. But for people with dementia, these normal changes are compounded in every way and are accompanied by other fundamental changes in how they think, speak, and act.

If you have been diagnosed with dementia, all of this will be painful and overwhelming to confront. This is why the first thing you need to do when you are diagnosed, the only thing you need to do, is allow yourself to experience your emotions. This will be different for every person, but this process is very likely to be similar to the stages of grief as defined by the psychiatrist Elisabeth Kübler-Ross: denial, anger, bargaining, depression, and, finally, acceptance. Give yourself the time and permission to experience and move through these emotions. If you need to feel angry, feel angry. If you need to feel depressed, feel depressed. Try not to lash out at others, but experience all the emotions it's natural to feel at this time. Try to talk to other people about how you feel and try not to isolate yourself, but at the same time, do what you need to do. Don't be ashamed of anything you feel right now. Your emotions are telling you what you need. Listen. There will be a time for understanding and for making important decisions, but that time is not when you are first diagnosed. This time is for you to figure out a way to confront this disease that seems most natural to you.

Once you have experienced the emotions you need to experience, then it is time to seek help to get some of the legal and financial documents you need in place. You won't want to think about this, but it is important to do now while you can still think clearly and make these important decisions for yourself. You can get help with this from your loved ones and learn the basics steps by reading *Long-Term Care Insurance, Power of Attorney, Wealth Management, and Other First Steps*. These first steps come with their own emotional struggles, and it's okay to embrace and experience those emotions, too. You're not alone in this, and whenever you need it, ask for help along the way.

The next two sections examine how to begin understanding the progression of dementia and coping with the diagnosis from the perspective of the individual with the disease. Then the following section turns to the caregiver to suggest ways that caregivers can help with that coping.

How Dementia Progresses

One thing that may help you if you have been diagnosed with dementia is to learn what the disease is and what it does. Probably the best way to approach understanding dementia is to learn what you should expect as the disease progresses. Although the effects of dementia and how it progresses are different for everyone who has it, generally people with dementia experience a gradual worsening of symptoms over time. In the early stages, memory loss and reduction of ability to function are minor and very gradual, but in the later phases, people with dementia lose the ability to participate in give-and-take conversation and react to stimuli. If you have dementia, activities you used to do easily, such as balancing a checkbook or keeping track of your keys, will become gradually more difficult. The checklist below focuses on the early changes to expect.

Checklist: Early changes to expect with dementia

☐ Disruptive memory loss, such as forgetting information you learned recently and important dates and events. You may ask for the same information again and again, but you may not remember that you've already asked for it.

☐ Difficulty solving problems, such planning an event and keeping track of bills. Working with numbers or following processes with many steps may become especially difficult.

☐ Being confused about time and place. You may have trouble remembering what day it is, why you are where you are and what you were doing, or what is happening right now.

- ☐ Misplacing things, such as not finding car keys where you expect them to be.

- ☐ Difficulty performing familiar work or personal tasks. This may make it challenging or impossible to continue working if you are not retired.

- ☐ Problems with self-expression, such as difficulty organizing thoughts or finding the right words to say what you mean. This may make it difficult for you to follow conversations or to take an active part in them.

- ☐ Impaired judgment that compromises decision making. This may be difficult for you to be aware of, but if you think you've paid for a good or service you haven't received, you notice charges that don't look right to you in your credit card statements, or you receive strange bills, ask for help from your caregivers in understanding what concerns you.

- ☐ Changes in mood and personality, such as depression, anxiety, or sudden and unpredictable irritability and anger. You may become socially withdrawn, even if you are normally very social, and you may lose motivation to complete tasks, especially challenging ones.

How to Cope if You Have Been Diagnosed with Dementia

If you feel embarrassed by your symptoms and are afraid to talk to others or ask for help, you are not alone. Many people with dementia experience this. However, trying to cover up the symptoms can be very stressful, and eventually it's impossible to cover up the signs. Instead, you should try to integrate changes from the disease into daily life while remaining as active and engaged as possible. If you have been diagnosed, remember to be flexible, fine-tune your approach from day to day, and ask for help. Although some people stigmatize the need to depend on others as weak and parasitic, it is wrong to view relationships this way, especially your relationships with close family and friends. People help one another not just out of a sense of obligation but also to find meaning and purpose in their own lives. If you let other people help you, you can better cope with the disease, and you may also help them cope better with it as well by giving them a way to deal with it. Remember: You and the ones who love and care for you are all in this together.

Checklist: How to cope with a diagnosis of dementia

- ☐ Research dementia and discuss your feelings and findings with loved ones.

- ☐ Involve family and friends in your efforts to learn all you can about dementia.

- ☐ Ask all medical providers to explain medical terms and instructions that you find confusing or do not remember. Encourage a close family member or friend to assist you in these efforts, helping you take note of anything important for you to know about your diagnosis.

☐ Find out what support services are available in your community. Local organizations may offer everything from transportation help to peer counseling.

☐ Decide who your primary caregivers should be and, with their help, begin creating and organizing a daily routine for yourself.

☐ If you feel overwhelmed with depression, anxiety, and stress following your diagnosis, don't hesitate to seek out a mental health provider. Meeting with a mental health professional early in the course of the disease can help you cope better as the condition worsens. For information on finding a mental health provider, see the Resources at the end of this book.

www.ingramcontent.com/pod-product-compliance
Lightning Source LLC
Chambersburg PA
CBHW060505280326
41933CB00014B/2864